AAOS

Bob Elling, MPA, REMT-P • Kirsten M. Elling, BS, REMT-P • Mikel A. Rothenberg, MD

Pathophysiology
Paramedic

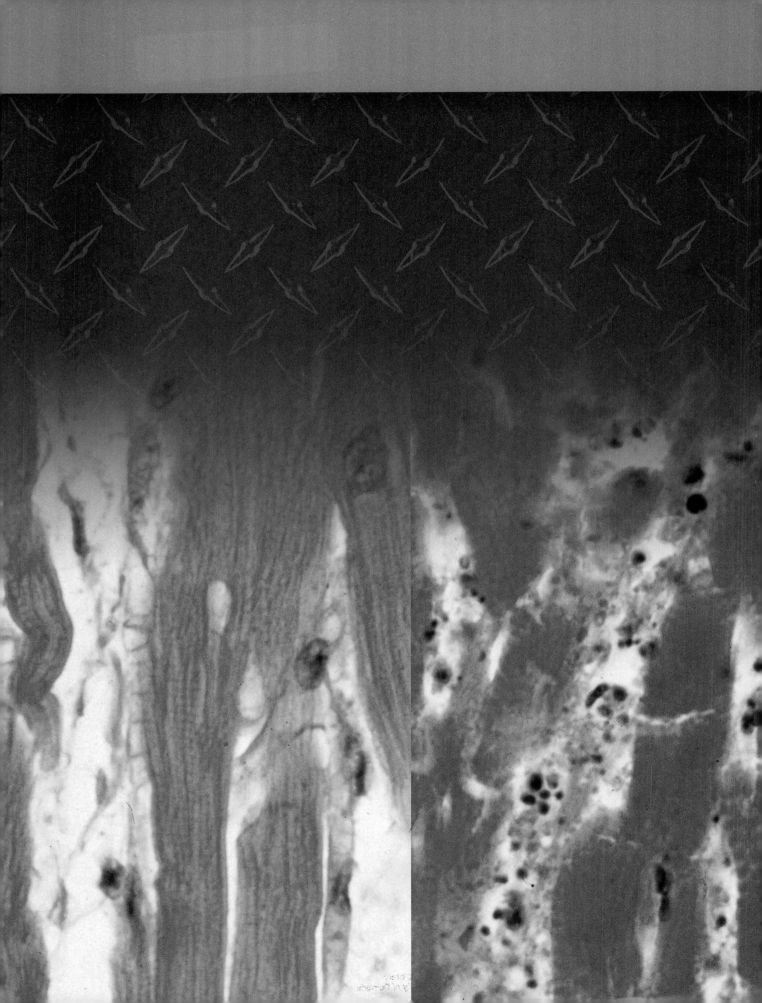

Pathophysiology
Paramedic

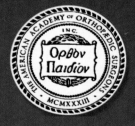

American Academy of Orthopaedic Surgeons

Andrew N. Pollak, MD, FAAOS
Editor
Medical Director, Baltimore County
Fire Department
Associate Professor, University
of Maryland School of Medicine
Baltimore, MD

Mikel A. Rothenberg, MD
EMS Educator
North Olmstead, OH

Bob Elling, MPA, REMT-P
Hudson Valley Community College
Andrew Jackson University
Colonie EMS Department
Schenectady, NY

Kirsten M. Elling, BS, REMT-P
Hudson Valley Community College
Colonie EMS Department
Schenectady, NY

JONES AND BARTLETT PUBLISHERS
Sudbury, Massachusetts
BOSTON   TORONTO   LONDON   SINGAPORE

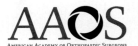

Jones and Bartlett Publishers

World Headquarters Jones and Bartlett Publishers
40 Tall Pine Drive, Sudbury, MA 01776
978-443-5000
info@jbpub.com
www.EMSzone.com

Production Credits
Chief Executive Officer: Clayton E. Jones
Chief Operating Officer: Donald W. Jones, Jr.
President, Higher Education and Professional Publishing: Robert W. Holland, Jr.
V.P., Sales and Marketing: William J. Kane
V.P., Production and Design: Anne Spencer
V.P., Manufacturing and Inventory Control: Therese Connell
Publisher, Public Safety: Kimberly Brophy
Editor: Christine Emerton
Production Editor: Karen Ferreira
Text Design: Studio Montage, Anne Spencer
Composition: Shepherd, Inc.
Cover Design: Kristin Ohlin
Printing and Binding: RR Donnelley/Kendallville

On the cover: Comparison of cardiac muscle fibers. Left: With necrotic fibers. Right: With fragmentation of fibers, loss of muscle staining, and fragmented bits of nuclear debris (original magnification, × 400).

Some images in this book feature models. These models do not necessarily endorse, represent, or participate in the activities represented in the images.

The procedures and protocols in this book are based on the most current recommendations of responsible medical sources. The American Academy of Orthopaedic Surgeons and the publisher, however, make no guarantee as to, and assume no responsibility for, the correctness, sufficiency, or completeness of such information or recommendations. Other or additional safety measures may be required under particular circumstances.

Editorial Credits
Chief Education Officer: Mark W. Wieting
Director, Department of Publications: Marilyn L. Fox, PhD
Managing Editor: Barbara A. Scotese

Jones and Bartlett's books and products are available through most bookstores and online booksellers. To contact Jones and Bartlett Publishers directly, call 800-832-0034, fax 978-443-8000, or visit our website www.jbpub.com.

Substantial discounts on bulk quantities of Jones and Bartlett's publications are available to corporations, professional associations, and other qualified organizations. For details and specific discount information, contact the special sales department at Jones and Bartlett via the above contact information or send an email to specialsales@jbpub.com.

This textbook is intended solely as a guide to the appropriate procedures to be employed when rendering emergency care to the sick and injured. It is not intended as a statement of the standard of care required in any particular situation, because circumstances and the patient's physical condition can vary widely from one emergency to another. Nor is it intended that this textbook shall in any way advise emergency personnel concerning legal authority to perform the activities or procedures discussed. Such local determinations should be made only with the aid of legal council.

Library of Congress Cataloging-in-Publication Data
Elling, Bob.
   Paramedic : pathophysiology / American Academy of Orthopaedic Surgeons ; Bob Elling, Kirsten M. Elling, Mikel A. Rothenberg ; editor Andrew N. Pollak.
      p. ; cm.
   Includes index.
   ISBN 0-7637-3765-8
   1. Physiology, Pathological—Outlines, syllabi, etc. 2. Allied health personnel—Outlines, syllabi, etc.
   [DNLM: 1. Pathology. 2. Allied Health Personnel. 3. Case Reports. 4. Disease Progression. 5. Inflammation. 6. Wounds and Injuries
QZ 4 E46p 2006] I. Elling, Kirsten M. II. Rothenberg, Mikel A. III. Pollak, Andrew N. IV. American Academy of Orthopaedic Surgeons. V. Title.
   RB113.E54 2006
   616.07—dc22

                              2005027721
6048

Additional credits appear on page 182, which constitutes a continuation of the copyright page.

Printed in the United States of America
17 16 15   10 9 8 7 6

Brief Contents

Table of Contents

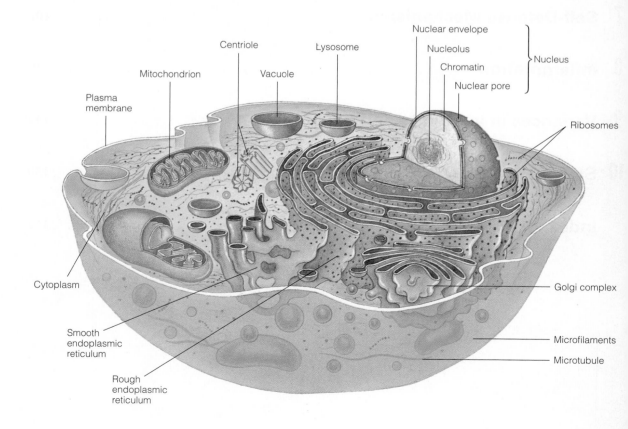

Chapter 5

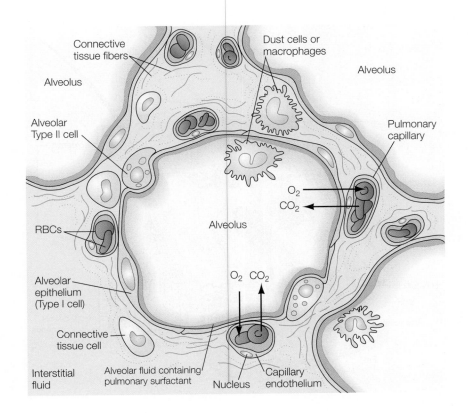

Connective tissue fibers

Dust cells or macrophages

Alveolus

Alveolus

Alveolar Type II cell

Pulmonary capillary

O_2

CO_2

RBCs

Alveolus

Alveolar epithelium (Type I cell)

O_2 CO_2

Connective tissue cell

Interstitial fluid

Alveolar fluid containing pulmonary surfactant

Nucleus

Capillary endothelium

Chapter 6

Chapter 7

Chapter 8

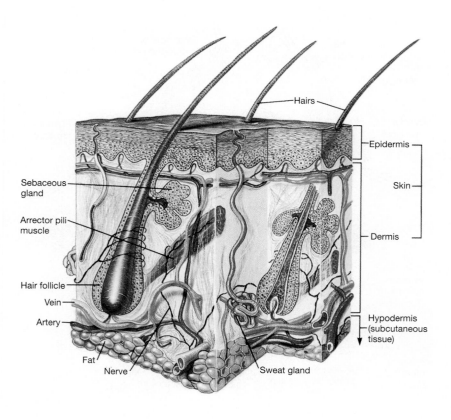

Hairs
Epidermis
Skin
Sebaceous gland
Dermis
Arrector pili muscle
Hair follicle
Vein
Artery
Hypodermis (subcutaneous tissue)
Fat
Nerve
Sweat gland

Chapter 9

Chapter 10

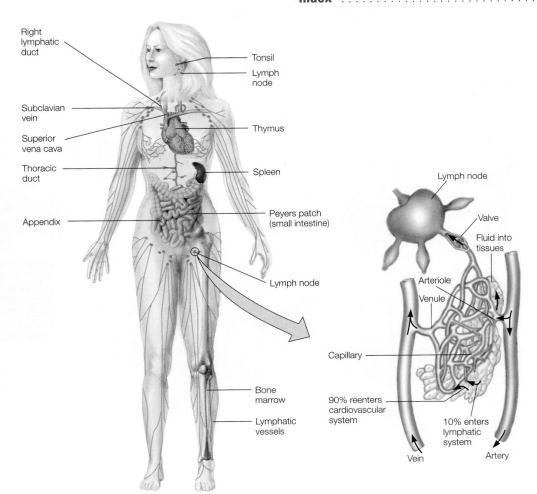

Resource Preview

Chapter Resources

Paramedic: Pathophysiology is designed to give paramedic professionals the education and confidence they need to effectively treat patients in the field. Features that will reinforce and expand on essential information include:

Navigation Toolbar

Found at the beginning of each chapter, the navigation toolbar will guide students through the technology resources and text features available for that chapter.

Self-Defense Mechanisms

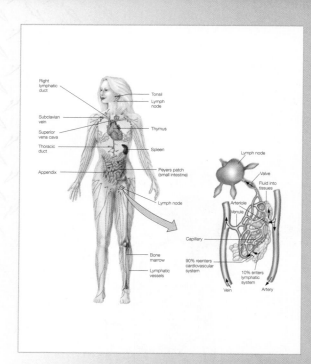

OBJECTIVES

Cognitive

1-6.13 Define the characteristics of the immune response. (p 108)

1-6.14 Discuss induction of the immune system. (p 113)

1-6.15 Discuss fetal and neonatal immune function. (p 120)

1-6.16 Discuss aging and the immune function in the elderly. (p 121)

Additional Objectives*

1. Summarize the humoral immune response. (p 115)

2. Summarize the cell-mediated immune response. (p 119)

3. Discuss interactions between innate and acquired immunity in bacterial infection. (p 120)

*These are noncurriculum objectives

www.Paramedic.EMSzone.com

Online Chapter Pretest
Vocabulary Explorer
Anatomy Review
Web Links

Case Studies
Physiology Tips
Medication Tips
Paramedic Safety Tips
Special Needs Tips
Vital Vocabulary
Prep Kit

Four-Color Illustrations

Highly descriptive, visually stunning images enable the paramedic to visualize physiologic processes and disease states.

Progressive Case Studies

Each chapter contains a progressive case study to make students start thinking about what they might do if they encountered a similar case in the field. The case study introduces patients and follows their progress from dispatch to delivery at the emergency department. The case becomes progressively more detailed as new material is presented. This feature, which includes additional diagnostic information, is a valuable learning tool that encourages critical thinking skills. Answers and rationales for the case study appear in the end of chapter Prep Kit.

---

8   Paramedic Pathophysiology

BODY SYSTEMS
Made up of cells organized by specialization to maintain homeostasis

Information from external environment relayed through nervous system

Nervous system
Acts through electrical signals to control rapid responses of the body; also responsible for higher functions—e.g., consciousness, memory, and creativity

Control

O_2

CO_2

Respiratory system
Obtains O_2 from, and eliminates CO_2, to external environment; helps regulate pH by adjusting the rate of removal of acid-forming CO_2

Urine containing wastes and excess water and ions

Urinary system
Removes wastes and excess water, salt, and other ions from the plasma and eliminates them in the urine; important in regulating the volume, ionic composition, and pH of the internal environment

Nutrients, water, ions

Digestive system
Obtains nutrients, water, and ions from the external environment and transfers them into the plasma; eliminates undigested food residues to external environment

Feces containing undigested food residues

Sperm enter female

Sperm leave male

Reproductive system
Not essential for homeostasis, but essential for perpetuation of species

External environment

Circulatory system
Transports nutrients, O_2, CO_2, wastes, ions, and hormones throughout body

Figure 1-4 The role of the body systems in maintaining homeostasis.

Physiology Tip

B lymphocytes originate from the same stem cells that give rise to all blood cell types. They mature in the bone marrow. T lymphocytes originate from the same bone marrow stem cells but travel to and mature in the thymus early in fetal life.

3. **Immune response:** The immune response is the body's defense reaction to any substance that is recognized as foreign. Often, this response is directed toward invading microbes, such as bacteria or viruses. However, the immune response is also triggered by foreign bodies (eg, a splinter) and even abnormal growths in our own cells (eg, a tumor).

Together, these three components of the immune system defend against foreign substances and disease-causing agents. Not all invaders can be destroyed by the body's immune system, however. In some cases, the best compromise the body can reach is to control the damage and keep the invader from spreading. Often, the immune system prevents severe disease following infection. When the normal systems become overwhelmed or fail, serious disease occurs.

Anatomy of the Immune System

The lymphatic system is a network of capillaries, vessels, ducts, nodes, and organs that help to maintain the fluid environment of the body by producing lymph and conveying it through the body (◄ Figure 7-1). The immune system has two anatomical components: the lymphoid tissues of the body and the cells that are responsible for the immune response.

Lymphoid tissues are distributed throughout the body. The two primary lymphoid tissues are the thymus gland and the bone marrow. Here cells involved in the immune response form and mature (► Figure 7-2). The thymus gland is a bilobed gland located below the thyroid gland and behind the sternum. It is prominent at birth and increases in size until the body reaches puberty. Then it becomes smaller and decreases in functional activity during adulthood. T lymphocytes originate from precursor cells in the bone marrow, leave the bone marrow, and mature in the thymus. The bone marrow is specialized soft tissue found within bone. Red bone marrow, widespread in the bones of children and found in some adult bones (eg, sternum, ribs), is essential for formation of mature blood cells. The bone marrow produces B lymphocytes.

In secondary lymphoid tissues, mature immune cells interact with invaders and initiate a response. Secondary tissues are divided into encapsulated tissues and unencapsulated diffuse lymphoid tissues. The encapsulated lymphoid tissues consist of the spleen and the lymph nodes. A lymph node (lymph gland) is a small structure that filters lymph and stores lymphocytes. Lymph nodes are concentrated in several areas of the body, such as the axillae, groin, and neck. The spleen is located on the left side of the body posterior and lateral to the stomach (left upper quadrant). This organ monitors the blood, destroys worn out red blood cells, and traps foreign invaders.

Case Study

Case Study, Part 1

Your unit is dispatched to a call for a severe allergic reaction from a bee sting. The dispatcher states that the patient is having difficulty breathing and that she gave herself an epinephrine auto-injection after being stung. When you arrive the patient is sitting up. Your general impression is that the patient is a young woman, about 28 years old, who is pale, sweating, and wheezing. She has blotches and hives on her neck and arms and her face looks swollen.

This patient is a high priority as her respiratory and circulatory systems are compromised. She is in anaphylactic shock. Her husband helped her with the epinephrine auto-injector, which was prescribed to her after the last time she was stung. The date on the injector indicates that it has not expired, and the syringe has been emptied.

Initial Assessment

Recording time
0 minutes

Appearance
Pale, sweaty, and unstable

Level of consciousness
Alert

Airway
Open

Vital Signs

Pulse rate/quality
140 beats/min, regular, weak

Blood pressure
80/40 mm Hg

Respiratory rate/depth
30 breaths/min, wheezing, shallow, and labored

Question 1: What is an antibody?

Question 2: What is an immune response?

Question 3: Describe the two general types of immune response.

CASE STUDY

Resource Preview

Paramedic Safety Tips

Serve to reinforce safety concerns for both the paramedic and the patient.

Medication Tips

Provide insight into the role of specific drugs.

---

38 · Paramedic Pathophysiology

Medication

Since pyrogens act by affecting the hypothalamic thermoregulatory center, fever-reducing drugs, such as aspirin or acetaminophen, are designed to blunt the hypothalamic response. Antipyretics inhibit the production of prostaglandins, which stimulate the hypothalamus, causing fever. By blocking these, antipyretics blunt the hypothalamic response.

Paramedic Safety

A significant exposure occurs when blood or body fluids come into contact with broken skin, the eyes, or other mucous membranes or through a parenteral (needle stick) contact. The most common virus that paramedics come into contact with in the field is hepatitis B, with 70,000 new infections reported annually in the United States. It is estimated that 500,000 Americans are currently infected with hepatitis, which causes inflammation of the liver. Always take body substance isolation precautions with all patients and have your personal protective equipment with you at all times. You should also always follow your agency's exposure control plan for the proper disposal of sharps.

reactions. The proliferation of microorganisms in the blood is called bacteremia, or sepsis.

Viral diseases are among the most common afflictions seen in humans. Viruses are intracellular parasites that take over the metabolic processes of the host cell and use the cell to help them replicate.

The protein coat that encapsulates most viruses protects them from phagocytosis. The replication of a virus inside the host cell because viruses do not contain any of their own organelles. Viral infection of a host cell leads to a decreased synthesis of macromolecules that are vital to the host cell (▶ Figure 3-6). As opposed to bacteria, viruses do not produce exotoxins or endotoxins.

There may be a symbiotic relationship between a virus and normal cells that results in a persistent unapparent infection. Viruses have been known to evoke a strong immune response and can rapidly produce an irreversible, lethal injury in highly susceptible cells, as is the case with acquired immunodeficiency syndrome (AIDS).

Immunologic and Inflammatory Injury

Inflammation is a protective response that can occur without bacterial invasion. Infection is the invasion of microorganisms that causes cell or tissue injury, which leads to the inflammatory response. The immune system provides protection for the body by providing defenses to attack and removing foreign organisms such as bacteria or viruses.

The cellular membranes may be injured by direct contact with the cellular and chemical components of the immune or inflammatory process such as phagocytes (lymphocytes and macrophages), histamine, antibodies, and lymphokines. When cell membranes are altered, potassium leaks out of the cells and water flows inward. The result is swelling of the cell. The nuclear envelope, organelle membranes, and the cell membrane may all rupture, leading to death of the cell. The degree of swelling and membrane rupture depends on the severity of the immune and inflammatory response.

Other Injurious Factors

Genetic factors, nutritional imbalances, and physical agents can also cause cell injury and death. Examples of injurious genetic factors affecting cells include chromosomal disorders (eg, Down syndrome), premature development of atherosclerosis, and obesity (some cases). There are two ways an abnormal gene may develop in an individual: (1) by mutation of the gene during meiosis, which affects the newly formed fetus, or (2) by heredity. In trisomy 21 (Down syndrome), the child is born with an extra chromosome, usually number 21.

Good nutrition is required to maintain good health and assist the cells in fighting off disease. Examples of nutritional disorders that can injure cells and the organism as a whole include obesity, malnutrition, vitamin excess or deficiency, and mineral excess or deficiency. Any of these conditions can lead to alterations in physical growth, mental and intellectual retardation, and even death in some circumstances.

Physical agents, such as heat, cold, and radiation, may cause cell injury. Examples include burns, frostbite, radiation sickness, and tumors. The degree of cell injury that results is determined by both the strength of the agent and the length of exposure.

---

50 · Paramedic Pathophysiology

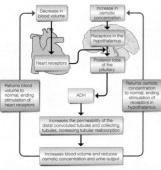

Figure 4-9 Antidiuretic hormone (ADH) secretion is under the control of the hypothalamus. When the osmotic concentration of the blood rises, receptors in the hypothalamus detect the change and trigger the release of ADH from the posterior lobe of the pituitary. Detectors in the heart also respond to changes in the blood volume. When it drops, they send signals to the brain, causing the release of ADH.

Physiology

When edematous tissue is compressed with a finger, the fluid is pushed aside causing an impression or "pit" that gradually refills. Referred to as pitting edema, this condition can be significant in patients who have chronic heart failure.

for these receptors are located primarily in the hypothalamus. When the extracellular fluid osmolarity is too high, they stimulate the production of ADH (see below).

2. Volume-sensitive receptors are receptors located in the atria that respond to stretch. When the intravascular fluid volume increases, the atria are stretched, leading to the release of natriuretic proteins (see below).

3. Baroreceptors are receptors found primarily in the carotid artery, aorta, and kidneys, which are sensitive to changes in the blood pressure.

The most potent stimulation for the release of ADH is an increase in blood osmolarity. Changes in blood volume and blood pressure are less of a stimulus. When osmolarity increases, the pituitary gland releases ADH, also known as vasopressin. ADH stimulates the kidneys to resorb water, decreasing the osmolarity of the blood.

Sodium and Chloride Balance

Sodium is the most common cation, or positively charged ion, in the body. The average adult has 60 mEq of sodium for each kilogram of body weight (2.2 lb = 1 kg). Most of the body's sodium is found in the extracellular fluid, but a small amount is found in the intracellular fluid. Intracellular sodium is transported out of the cell by the sodium-potassium pump because a resting cell membrane is relatively impermeable to sodium. Sodium also plays an important role in the regulation of the body's acid-base balance (sodium bicarbonate buffer system).

Sodium is taken in with foods. As little as 500 mg/d meets the body's needs. In the United States, studies have shown that the average adult

Physiology Tips

Tie concepts into practice.

Vital Vocabulary

Key terms are easily identified and defined.
A comprehensive list follows each chapter.

Special Needs Tips

Serve to highlight specific concerns for the elderly
and/or pediatric patient.

Prep Kit

End of chapter resources reinforce important concepts
with a chapter summary, comprehensive list of vital
vocabulary, and case study answers and rationales.

---

102   **Paramedic Pathophysiology**

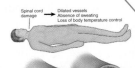

Spinal cord damage → Dilated vessels
Absence of sweating
Loss of body temperature control

Normal vessel   Dilated vessel

Figure 6-7 Damage to the spinal cord can cause significant injury to the part of the nervous system that controls the size and muscle tone of blood vessels. If the muscles in the blood vessels are cut off from their impulses to contract, then the vessels dilate widely, increasing the size and capacity of the vascular system. The blood in the body can no longer fill the enlarged vessels, resulting in inadequate perfusion in the form of neurogenic shock.

Multiple Organ Dysfunction Syndrome

Multiple organ dysfunction syndrome (MODS) is a progressive condition usually characterized by com-

Special Needs Tip

In children, the immune system is not fully developed; on the other hand, the geriatric patient experiences decreased immune function as part of the normal aging process. As a result, both patient groups have an increased susceptibility to infection. This in turn is a common cause of MODS. The organs of the very old or very young patient have a limited physiologic reserve. Thus when organs begin to fail, serious problems are evident fairly early in the process.

which is a potent vasodilator. Vasodilation leads to tissue hypoperfusion and may also contribute to hypotension.

The net outcome of activation of the above systems is maldistribution of both the systemic and organ blood flow. Often tissues attempt to compensate by accelerating their metabolism. The result is an oxygen supply–demand imbalance with tissue hypoxia and includes:

• Tissue hypoperfusion
• Exhaustion of the cells' fuel supply (adenosine triphosphate)

Prep Kit

Chapter Summary

• Pathophysiology is the study of how normal physiological processes can be altered by disease or the body's response to injury.
• Cells communicate electrochemically through a process called cell signaling. Cells signal through the release of hormones that bind to proteins called receptors, located on the surface of the receiving cells. This signaling triggers chemical reactions that lead to biological action in the receiving cells.
• Homeostasis, or the dynamic steady state in health, exists due to a balance between opposing normal regulatory systems.
• Ligands are molecules, whether produced by the body (endogenous) or given as a drug (exogenous), that bind a receptor, causing an action to occur. Ligands include electrolytes, neurotransmitters, and hormones and bind receptors leading to chemical reactions in cells to provide feedback inhibition.
• When abnormal cell signaling occurs, disease results. This is because alterations in cell signaling disrupt normal feedback processes leading to unopposed positive or inappropriate negative signaling and resultant disease states.

Vital Vocabulary

<u>autocrine hormone</u> A hormone that acts on the cell that secretes it.

<u>cell signaling</u> The process by which cells communicate with one another.

<u>counter-regulatory systems</u> Systems that consist of an opposing function for every function.

<u>dynamic steady state</u> Another term or description for homeostasis.

<u>endocrine hormones</u> Hormones that are carried to their target or cell group in the bloodstream.

<u>exocrine hormones</u> Hormones that are secreted through ducts into an organ or onto epithelial surfaces.

<u>feedback inhibition</u> Negative feedback resulting in the decrease of an action in the body.

<u>homeostasis</u> A term derived from the Greek words for "same" and "steady." All organisms constantly adjust their physiological processes in an effort to maintain an internal balance.

<u>hormones</u> Proteins formed in specialized organs or glands and carried to another organ or group of cells in the same organism. Hormones regulate many body functions, including metabolism, growth, and temperature.

<u>ligand</u> Any molecule that binds a receptor leading to a reaction.

<u>negative feedback</u> The concept that once the desired effect of a process has been achieved, further action is inhibited until it is needed again; also called feedback inhibition.

<u>neurotransmitters</u> Proteins that transmit signals between cells of the nervous system.

<u>normal regulatory systems</u> All normal body processes.

<u>paracrine hormones</u> Hormones that diffuse through intracellular spaces to their target.

<u>pathophysiology</u> The study of how normal physiological processes are altered by disease.

<u>positive feedback</u> A signal within a feedback loop that causes an action within that loop to increase.

Case Study Answers

Question 1: What do you suspect is the cause of this patient's confusion?

Answer: Systemic hypothermia would be high on the list but you still need to suspect other causes of altered mental status, such as stroke, transient ischemic attack, head injury, diabetes, hypoxia, and seizure.

Question 2: What additional assessment or diagnostic tools should you consider using with this patient?

Answer: On the basis of the patient's cold skin and history of diabetes, it would be appropriate to obtain a tympanic temperature (because he might have a low body temperature) and obtain a few drops of blood for a determination of the patient's level of blood glucose (since he has a history of diabetes).

Question 3: What is the significance of the patient's uncontrollable shivering?

Answer: Shivering is a normal compensatory mechanism that the body uses to create heat. It is a good sign that the body is trying to bring its temperature back to the normal range. A lack of shivering might indicate that the hypothermia is so severe that his body's thermoregulatory mechanism has already failed.

Question 4: Which homeostatic mechanism has been affected by the prolonged exposure to the cold?

Answer: The homeostatic mechanism that has been affected is the body's thermometer, which is called thermoregulation. The body normally maintains its temperature at a steady 98.6°F, or 37.0°C. Thermoregulation has one of the major roles of the metabolic process. The body's metabolism generates body heat and requires fuel (food) to burn, just as a furnace needs fuel to heat. In addition to the exposure to cold, the patient had not eaten and thus had low fuel reserves.

Question 5: What are the potential causes of the patient's altered mental status?

Answer: The patient's glucose reading is low at 60 mg/dL. The normal range is 80 to 120 mg/dL. Low levels of blood glucose can cause confusion and unconsciousness, and, if not treated promptly, coma and death. There are many reasons that a patient can have an altered mental status. Consider causes such as head injury, seizure, stroke or transient ischemic attack, hypoxia, electrolyte imbalance, ECG abnormality, hypothermia or hyperthermia, an overdose of drugs or alcohol, and complications of diabetes. The patient's altered mental status in this case is most likely a combination of low blood glucose levels and hypothermia.

Question 6: Now that you have learned more about this patient's medical history, what do you suspect?

Answer: The cold outside temperature combined with the patient's history of diabetes and lack of eating a scheduled meal quickly exhausted his energy reserves and his ability to produce body heat. With the onset of confusion, the patient was unable to seek help and became colder and more confused.

Question 7: By observing the patient's response to the treatment provided, which condition, hypothermia or hypoglycemia (low blood glucose level), is quicker to reverse?

Answer: When the brain gets the sugar it needs through intake of food or IV, the body responds quickly. Raising the body's temperature is a slow process, and it must be accomplished slowly to prevent an adverse reaction. In the emergency department this can be done by warming up the core of the body with warm inhaled oxygen, warm IV fluids, specialty blankets, heating lamps, and more aggressive maneuvers such as heart-lung bypass and dialysis.

CASE STUDY ANSWERS

www.Paramedic.EMSzone.com

Resource Preview

Instructor Resources

Instructor's ToolKit CD-ROM

ISBN: 0-7637-4203-1

Preparing for class is easy with the resources found on this CD-ROM, including:

- **PowerPoint Presentations**   Providing you with a powerful way to make presentations that are educational and engaging to your students. The slides can be edited and modified to meet your needs.

- **Lecture Outlines**   Providing you with complete ready-to-use lesson plans that outline all of the topics covered in the text. The lesson plans can be modified and customized to fit your needs.

- **Image Bank**   Providing you with a selection of images found in the text. You can use them to incorporate more images into the PowerPoint presentation, make handouts, or enlarge a specific image for further discussion.

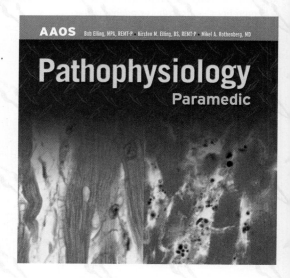

The resources on the Instructor's ToolKit CD-ROM that accompanies this text have been formatted so that instructors can seamlessly integrate them into the most popular course administration tools. Please feel free to contact Jones and Bartlett technical support at any time with questions.

Technology Resources

- **Web Links**   Present current information, including trends in paramedic care and new equipment.

- **Online Chapter Pretests**   Prepare students for training with instant results and feedback on incorrect answers.

- **Vocabulary Explorer**   Interactive online glossary to expand student's medical vocabulary.

- **Animated Flash Cards**   Review vital vocabulary and key concepts.

- **Anatomy Review**   Interactive anatomic figure labeling.

www.Paramedic.EMSzone.com

Acknowledgments

Reviewers

John Gosford, EMT-P
Tallahassee, FL

Brent Ricks, MS, REMT-P
Hudson Valley Community College
Troy, NY

Jonathan S. Halpert, MD, FACEP, REMT-P
St Peter's Hospital
Albany, NY

Anthony Cuda, NREMT-P
Community College of Allegheny County
Pittsburgh, PA

Joseph L. Brown, Jr., EMT-P
Baltimore County Fire Department
Towson, MD

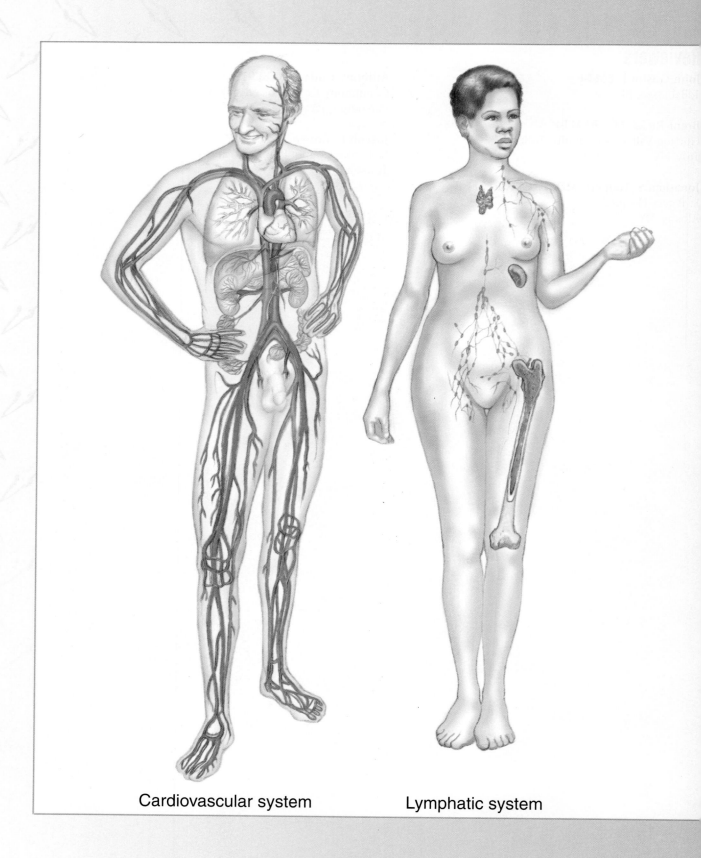

Cardiovascular system   Lymphatic system

Pathophysiology: What, Why, and How
It Is Important to the Paramedic

OBJECTIVES

Cognitive

1-6.26 Describe homeostasis as a dynamic steady state. (p 4–5)

Affective

1-6.31 Advocate the need to understand and apply the knowledge of pathophysiology to patient assessment and treatment. (p 4)

Additional Objectives*

1. Define pathophysiology. (p 4)

2. Describe the role of feedback inhibition (negative feedback) in maintenance of homeostasis. (p 5)

3. List the differences between endocrine, exocrine, and paracrine hormones. (p 6)

4. Discuss how loss of normal cell signaling leads to positive feedback and disease. (p 7)

5. Explain how the understanding of pathophysiology is helpful to the paramedic in the field. (p 4)

*These are noncurriculum objectives.

www.Paramedic.EMSzone.com

TECHNOLOGY

- Online Chapter Pretest
- Vocabulary Explorer
- Anatomy Review
- Web Links

Chapter FEATURES

- Case Studies
- Physiology Tips
- Medication Tips
- Paramedic Safety Tips
- Special Needs Tips
- Vital Vocabulary
- Prep Kit

Pathophysiology

<u>Pathophysiology</u> is the study of how normal physiological processes can be altered by disease or the body's response to injury. Essentially, pathophysiology delineates the mechanisms of disease processes. Understanding disease processes is important for paramedics to anticipate situations better, correct problems, and provide the most appropriate care to their patients. Once you understand the physical laws and basics of normal body function, applying them to the mechanisms and complications of disease is straightforward.

Homeostasis—The Dynamic Steady State

Originally described by Walter B. Cannon in 1932, <u>homeostasis</u> is a term derived from the Greek words for "same" and "steady." All organisms constantly adjust their physiological processes in an effort to maintain an internal balance. This balance or effort to maintain the same steady environment through the use of internal automatic mechanisms is called homeostasis. Homeostasis is the foundation of all normal body processes, also termed <u>normal regulatory systems</u>. An example of a homeostatic mechanism would be the body's control of its internal temperature despite the fluctuations in the external temperature. All body components, from the smallest cell to the largest organ system, constantly communicate with one another to maintain the critical balance required for health. There is a physiological balance within the organism. Thus, for every cell, tissue, or organ system that performs one function, there is always at least one that performs an opposing function. For example, the autonomic

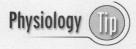

Physiology Tip

A useful metaphor for homeostasis is the Taoist symbol of yin-yang—a circle with two equal and opposite halves, one black and one white. This symbol of the Tai Chi philosophy represents the balance of opposites, or the positive and negative aspects of nature. According to this philosophy, the balance of yin and yang reflects wholeness and essential balance. So too with the human body: For every body system that performs one function, there is always at least one other that performs an opposing function so that equilibrium can be maintained.

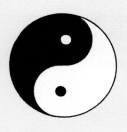

nervous system consists of the sympathetic and parasympathetic components, which act to speed up or slow down the activity of target organs. Systems that provide this counterbalance are often called <u>counter-regulatory systems</u>. The communication and interaction between these opposing normal regulatory systems allows for maintenance of the status quo, or steady state. Because homeostasis

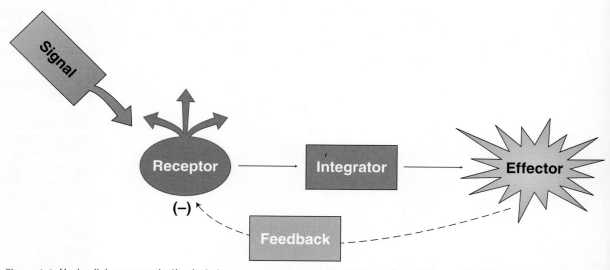

Figure 1-1 Most cellular communication includes a component of negative feedback in which the product of a reaction feeds back to its own "assembly line," stopping its own production.

efers to active processes, it is sometimes called the **dynamic steady state**. Knowledge of the coordination of specific body functions leads to a better understanding of disease processes.

Examples of homeostatic mechanisms include the body's regulation of temperature, the regulation of pH or the acid-base balance, and the balance of water or hydration status of the body.

Cell Signaling and Feedback

Most communication within the body takes place at the cellular level. Cells communicate electrochemically through a process called **cell signaling**. Cells signal through the release of molecules (such as hormones) that bind to proteins called *receptors,* located on the surface of the receiving cells. This signaling triggers chemical reactions in the receiving cells that lead to a biological action. When the action is completed, the opposing system steps in, "turning off" the action. Biologically, this cessation is termed **feedback inhibition** or **negative feedback**. Most cellular communication includes a component of negative feedback in which the product of a reaction feeds information back to its own "assembly line," stopping its own production (◄ Figure 1-1).

The thermostat mechanism in a home is a good example of a feedback mechanism. Consider your home in the middle of the winter. Heat is constantly being lost through the windows, doors, and any poorly insulated areas. The thermostat detects the decrease in temperature and signals the furnace to produce heat to rewarm the house. Once the temperature rises past a selected point, the thermostat gives feedback to the furnace to shut down to prevent overheating. This feedback process keeps the house temperature within a selected range (► Figure 1-2). As you learned in your EMT-B training, the body is constantly generating heat through its cellular processes, and there are five primary mechanisms that help the body eliminate excess temperature or heat—convection, conduction, radiation, evaporation, and respiration. The body's thermostat works to balance the generation of heat with the processes of heat elimination. This complex process is an example of the homeostatic balance in the body.

The human body maintains homeostasis by balancing what it takes in with what it puts out. For example, the body takes in chemicals and electrolytes, sugars, food, and water. It utilizes the nutrients, proteins, sugars, and oxygen and then eliminates the unnecessary chemicals and byproducts through respiration (carbon dioxide), urine and sweat (excess liquids), and feces (solid waste). ► Figure 1-3 illustrates the human body in this normal balance.

Case Study

CASE STUDY

Case Study, Part 1

Your unit is dispatched to a private residence on the outskirts of town on a cold winter day. After establishing that the scene is safe, you are met at the door by a woman. She states that her 72-year-old father was letting the dog out when he accidentally locked himself out of the house. She suspects that he may have been wandering around the backyard in his pajamas for the past 3 hours while she was out shopping. The temperature is approximately 22°F. The patient, who is seated at the kitchen table, is sitting quietly and appears to be shivering uncontrollably. He is covered in a heavy blanket, and a cup of hot tea and an uneaten lunch are on the table. The patient knows his name but is not sure of the day of the week or his exact location. His airway is open, and he is breathing rapidly. His circulatory status is stable, with a pulse and no obvious external bleeding although his skin is pale, cold to the touch, and dry. The patient's daughter tells you he has diabetes. You determine that ALS will be needed.

Initial Assessment

Recording time
0 minutes

Appearance
Shivering, pale, and dry

Level of consciousness
Verbal: knows his name but confused about where he is and how long he was outside

Airway
Open and clear

Vital Signs

Pulse rate/quality
60 beats/min, regular, and weak

Blood pressure
140/70 mm Hg

Respiratory rate/depth
24 breaths/min and shallow

Question 1: What do you suspect is the cause of this patient's confusion?

Question 2: What additional assessment or diagnostic tools should you consider using with this patient?

Question 3: What is the significance of the patient's uncontrollable shivering?

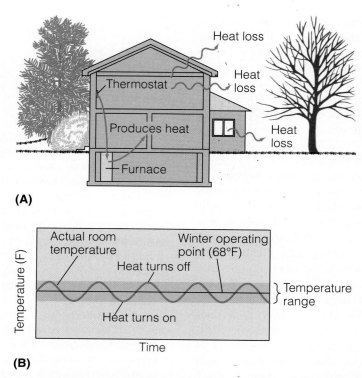

(A)

(B)

Figure 1-2 Homeostasis and the house. **A.** Heat is maintained in a house by a furnace, which compensates for heat loss. The thermostat monitors the internal temperature and switches the furnace on and off in response to temperature changes. **B.** A hypothetical temperature graph showing temperature fluctuation around the operating point.

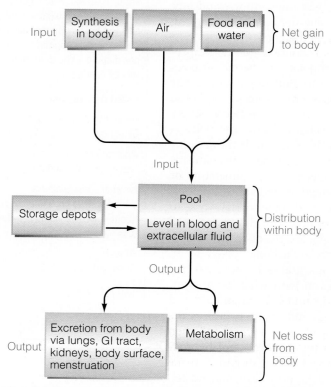

Figure 1-3 Generalized view of a homeostatic system. Inputs and outputs are balanced to maintain more or less constant levels of chemical and physical parameters.

Excessive output can rapidly upset homeostasis (eg, severe diarrhea kills millions of children each year in some nations; severe perspiration can cause excessive water loss and dehydration). Changes in input can also rapidly upset homeostasis (eg, going without water for 3 or more days can be life threatening; excess intake of salt can cause hypertension in some patients). Each of the body's systems serves a role in maintaining homeostasis (▶ Figure 1-4).

The degree of fluid imbalance required to alter homeostasis and result in illness depends on the patient's size, age, and underlying medical conditions. In healthy adults, loss of more than 30% of total body fluid is required, but a loss of only 10% to 15% of total body fluid in a small child could easily result in symptoms. Fluid therapy in appropriate patients is part of the basics of resuscitation—airway, breathing, and circulation. Fluid therapy, based on local protocols, should be administered in symptomatic patients.

Ligands and Receptors

A <u>ligand</u> is *any molecule*, whether produced by the body (endogenous) or given as a drug (exogenous) that binds *any receptor, anywhere*, leading to *any reaction*. Besides drugs given to a person, other common ligands include hormones, neurotransmitters, and electrolytes. <u>Hormones</u> are substances formed in very small amounts in one specialized organ or group of cells and carried to another organ or group of cells in the same organism. Hormones perform specific regulatory actions. <u>Endocrine hormones</u> are carried to their target organ or cell group in the blood. Examples include thyroid hormones and adrenal steroids. <u>Exocrine hormones</u> reach their target via a specific duct that opens into an organ. Examples of exocrine secretions are stomach acids

Medication Tip

Cell signaling and ligand-receptor interactions are currently one of the "hottest" research areas in medicine. A substantial number of diseases are evidence of an abnormality in cellular communication. A common example is cancer. Tumors result from cells that have grown out of control, usually because they do not respond to normal regulatory signals that tell them when to die off or stop proliferating. New research efforts are being directed toward repairing the abnormal communication link, either with chemotherapy, gene therapy, or stem cells.

Case Study

Case Study, Part 2

You discover that the patient has some nausea and continues to be confused. He has difficulty concentrating and his answers are inappropriate. The focused physical exam reveals a thin older man with clear lung sounds and a slight weakness on his right side. His speech is slightly slurred, but his daughter mentions that he often sounds that way, especially early in the morning or when his "sugar" is off. His hands and feet are cold and blue, and you suspect that his feet have frostbite. As you ask the daughter about the remainder of the SAMPLE history, you learn that her father is under the care of an endocrinologist for his diabetes and has a history of hypertension. As a type II diabetic who developed the disease in later life, he takes chlorpropamide (a diabetic agent) to control his blood sugar. He takes hydrochlorothiazide (an antihypertensive drug) to control his blood pressure and also takes an aspirin a day because he had a transient ischemic attack, or mini-stroke, 2 years ago.

You administer oxygen to the patient and take his temperature. You also decide to do a finger stick to check his blood glucose level. You begin treatment by administering oxygen via a nonrebreathing mask and by removing any wet clothing. You carefully wrap and splint both of his feet and place him onto a stretcher, wrapping him in wool blankets. You move him to the ambulance and begin transport to the hospital.

Focused Physical Assessment

Recording time
10 minutes

Appearance
Continues to shiver

Lung sounds
Clear in all fields

Skin signs
Pale, distal extremities are cold and blue
No peripheral edema or jugular vein distention

Diagnostic Tools

SpO_2
94%

Blood glucose level
60 mg/dL

Electrocardiogram
Bradycardia with occasional unifocal premature ventricular contractions

Tympanic temperature
95°F

Question 4: Which homeostatic mechanism has been affected by the prolonged exposure to the cold?

Question 5: What are the potential causes of the patient's altered mental status?

CASE STUDY

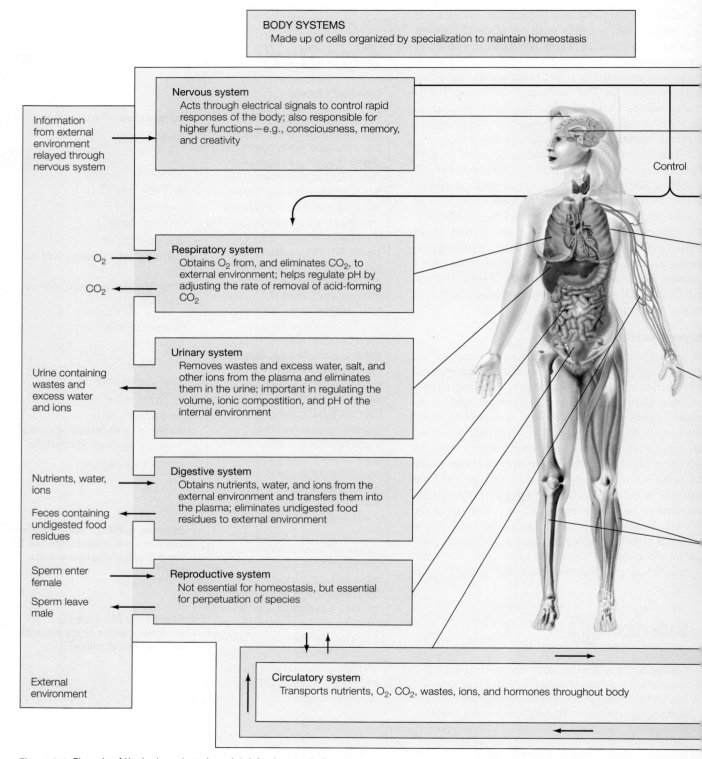

BODY SYSTEMS
Made up of cells organized by specialization to maintain homeostasis

Nervous system
Acts through electrical signals to control rapid responses of the body; also responsible for higher functions—e.g., consciousness, memory, and creativity

Information from external environment relayed through nervous system

Control

Respiratory system
Obtains O_2 from, and eliminates CO_2, to external environment; helps regulate pH by adjusting the rate of removal of acid-forming CO_2

O_2

CO_2

Urinary system
Removes wastes and excess water, salt, and other ions from the plasma and eliminates them in the urine; important in regulating the volume, ionic compostition, and pH of the internal environment

Urine containing wastes and excess water and ions

Digestive system
Obtains nutrients, water, and ions from the external environment and transfers them into the plasma; eliminates undigested food residues to external environment

Nutrients, water, ions

Feces containing undigested food residues

Reproductive system
Not essential for homeostasis, but essential for perpetuation of species

Sperm enter female

Sperm leave male

External environment

Circulatory system
Transports nutrients, O_2, CO_2, wastes, ions, and hormones throughout body

Figure 1-4 The role of the body systems in maintaining homeostasis.

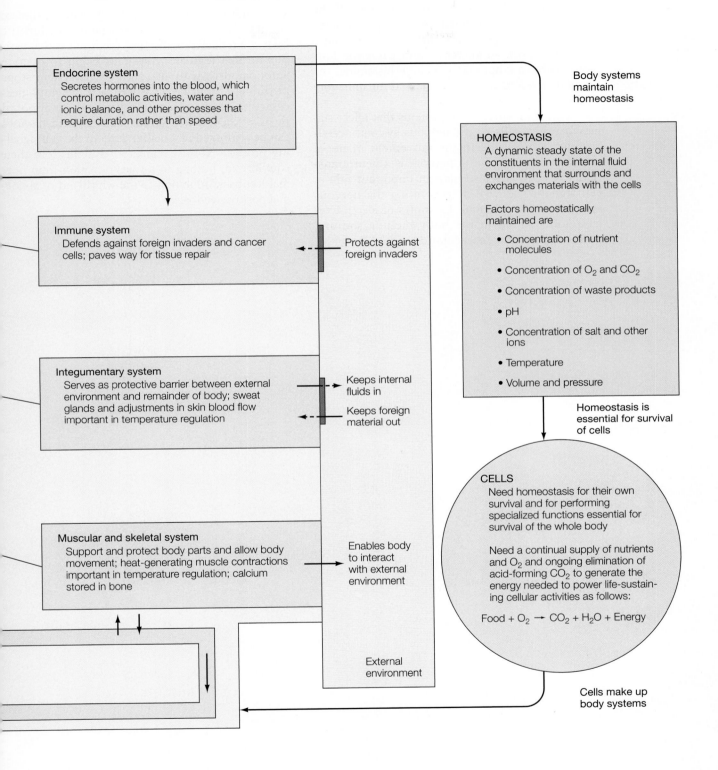

Endocrine system
Secretes hormones into the blood, which control metabolic activities, water and ionic balance, and other processes that require duration rather than speed

Immune system
Defends against foreign invaders and cancer cells; paves way for tissue repair

Protects against foreign invaders

Integumentary system
Serves as protective barrier between external environment and remainder of body; sweat glands and adjustments in skin blood flow important in temperature regulation

Keeps internal fluids in

Keeps foreign material out

Muscular and skeletal system
Support and protect body parts and allow body movement; heat-generating muscle contractions important in temperature regulation; calcium stored in bone

Enables body to interact with external environment

External environment

Body systems maintain homeostasis

HOMEOSTASIS
A dynamic steady state of the constituents in the internal fluid environment that surrounds and exchanges materials with the cells

Factors homeostatically maintained are

- Concentration of nutrient molecules

- Concentration of O_2 and CO_2

- Concentration of waste products

- pH

- Concentration of salt and other ions

- Temperature

- Volume and pressure

Homeostasis is essential for survival of cells

CELLS
Need homeostasis for their own survival and for performing specialized functions essential for survival of the whole body

Need a continual supply of nutrients and O_2 and ongoing elimination of acid-forming CO_2 to generate the energy needed to power life-sustaining cellular activities as follows:

$$Food + O_2 \rightarrow CO_2 + H_2O + Energy$$

Cells make up body systems

and perspiration. <u>Paracrine hormones</u> diffuse through intracellular spaces to their target. If the hormone acts on the cell that secreted it, it is called an <u>autocrine hormone</u>. In some cases, a substance may act as both an autocrine and paracrine hormone. Paracrine hormones include histamine, the hormone released during allergic and inflammatory reactions.

<u>Neurotransmitters</u> are proteins that affect signals between cells of the nervous system; acetylcholine, which aids in the movement of nerve impulses from neuron to neuron, is a neurotransmitter. Electrolytes also play an important role in cell signaling as well as generating the nervous system's action potential. Examples of electrolytes commonly found in the body include sodium, potassium, calcium, and chloride.

Abnormal Cell Signaling and Disease

When normal cell signaling is interrupted, disease occurs. The normal counterbalances within the body are rendered ineffective; the result is that various normal regulatory systems begin to operate autonomously, without control. The system stops providing critical negative feedback, which is necessary to regulate function; instead, unopposed <u>positive feedback</u> is given. Many human diseases can be attributed to a malfunction in the cell signaling process. Normal regulatory systems lose their equilibrium, leading to a transformation from normal feedback inhibition to the whirlwind of abnormal positive feedback.

Physiology Tip

In heart failure, the kidneys are hypoperfused by a poorly contracting heart. As a result, volume and pressure sensors in the kidneys "think" the patient is hypovolemic and hypotensive; in response, the body produces the hormone angiotensin II, causing salt and water retention and vasoconstriction. If the patient were truly hypotensive and hypovolemic, both actions of the angiotensin II would be beneficial to the patient. However, the patient in heart failure is actually *fluid over-loaded*. Unfortunately, due to this lack of cell signaling between the actual intravascular volume and the kidneys, the patient continues to produce angiotensin II; this in effect worsens the heart failure through continued fluid retention. As long as heart failure continues with hypoperfusion of the kidneys, the cycle persists.

Case Study

Case Study, Part 3

The heater in the ambulance is turned up to high. The patient is given warm IV fluids and high concentration glucose through the IV line. During transport, you perform an ongoing assessment of the patient. The patient's mental status is improving slowly and the shivering is less intense. He understands that he is being taken to the hospital. His vital signs show a slight improvement with a stronger pulse and improved respiratory effort.

Ongoing Assessment

Recording Time
25 minutes

Appearance
Less shivering

Mental status
Slowly improving

Skin signs
Not as pale as previously noted, distal extremities still cold and blue

Vital Signs

Pulse rate/quality
68 beats/min, regular, and stronger

Blood pressure
138/70 mm Hg

Respiratory rate/depth
20 breaths/min and regular

Diagnostics

SpO2
98%

Blood glucose level
144 mg/dL

Electrocardiogram
Normal sinus rhythm at 68 beats/min

Question 6: Now that you have learned more about this patient's medical history, what do you suspect?

Question 7: By observing the patient's response to the treatment provided, which condition, hypothermia or hypoglycemia (low blood glucose level), is quicker to reverse?

Case Study

Case Study, Part 4

Completion of the Case Study

While en route to the hospital, you call hospital personnel to advise them of your patient. As the patient's condition is stable and steadily improving, you do not request any further medication or special procedures.

After you transfer the patient to hospital personnel, you talk to the patient's daughter and offer a suggestion to help prevent this from occurring again. You suggest subscribing to a "lifeline-type" service, in which the patient can trigger an alarm when he feels he needs some assistance. She thanks you for all your help.

Paramedic Safety Tip

The respiratory process is actually a feedback loop that continues to work throughout our lifetime. We constantly exchange gases with the environment: We breathe in oxygen that our circulatory system transports to every cell in the body and then exhale the cellular waste product carbon dioxide. This loop effectively regulates our blood's oxygen and carbon dioxide levels, provided the environment is stable (▼ **Figure 1-5**). However, the respiratory feedback loop can be interrupted, for example, by inhaling pollutants or dangerous gases or chemicals. Paramedics often are called to treat patients who have been exposed to chemicals by inhalation, most commonly carbon monoxide. When exposed to carbon monoxide, sulfur oxides, nitrogen oxides, or vehicle exhaust, fires, and cigarette smoke, the body's blood chemistry changes along with respiratory system functioning, increasing respiratory

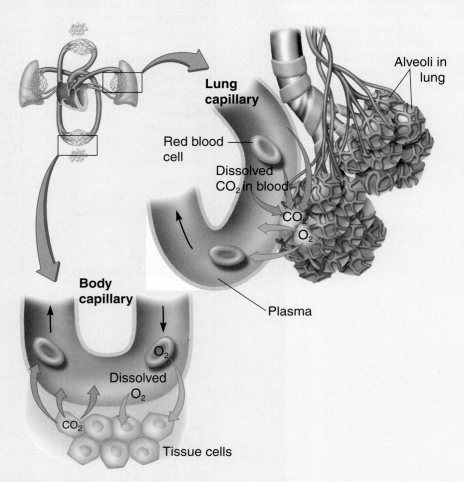

Figure 1-5 Breathing as a feedback loop.

symptoms and disease. Examples may include the long-term lung damage that occurs due to second-hand smoke or working in hazardous environments such as coal mines or asbestos removal (▼ Figure 1-6). If you come in contact with fires or toxic inhalants in the course of your work as a paramedic, be sure to always wear your personal protective equipment and self-contained breathing apparatus as appropriate!

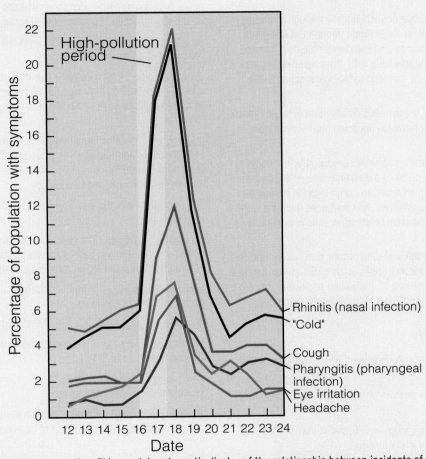

Figure 1-6 The pollution connection. This graph is a dramatic display of the relationship between incidents of respiratory illnesses and an episode of high air pollution in New York City in 1962. In a 2-day period—days 16 and 17—sulfur dioxide levels rose from 0.2 ppm to 0.8-0.9 ppm, and immediately the numbers of nasal infections, colds, coughs, pharyngeal infections, eye irritation, and headaches all rose dramatically. Adapted from McCarroll JR, et al, Health and the urban environment: Health profiles versus environmental pollutants. *Am J Public Health*. 1966;56:266-275.

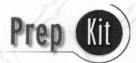

Chapter Summary

- Pathophysiology is the study of how normal physiological processes can be altered by disease or the body's response to injury.

- Cells communicate electrochemically through a process called cell signaling. Cells signal through the release of hormones that bind to proteins called receptors, located on the surface of the receiving cells. This signaling triggers chemical reactions that lead to biological action in the receiving cells.

- Homeostasis, or the dynamic steady state in health, exists due to a balance between opposing normal regulatory systems.

- Ligands are molecules, whether produced by the body (endogenous) or given as a drug (exogenous), that bind a receptor, causing an action to occur. Ligands include electrolytes, neurotransmitters, and hormones and bind receptors leading to chemical reactions in cells to provide feedback inhibition.

- When abnormal cell signaling occurs, disease results. This is because alterations in cell signaling disrupt normal feedback processes leading to unopposed positive or inappropriate negative signaling and resultant disease states.

Vital Vocabulary

autocrine hormone A hormone that acts on the cell that secretes it.

cell signaling The process by which cells communicate with one another.

counter-regulatory systems Systems that consist of an opposing function for every function.

dynamic steady state Another term or description for homeostasis.

endocrine hormones Hormones that are carried to their target or cell group in the bloodstream.

exocrine hormones Hormones that are secreted through ducts into an organ or onto epithelial surfaces.

feedback inhibition Negative feedback resulting in the decrease of an action in the body.

homeostasis A term derived from the Greek words for "same" and "steady." All organisms constantly adjust their physiological processes in an effort to maintain an internal balance.

hormones Proteins formed in specialized organs or glands and carried to another organ or group of cells in the same organism. Hormones regulate many body functions, including metabolism, growth, and temperature.

ligand Any molecule that binds a receptor leading to a reaction.

negative feedback The concept that once the desired effect of a process has been achieved, further action is inhibited until it is needed again; also called feedback inhibition.

neurotransmitters Proteins that transmit signals between cells of the nervous system.

normal regulatory systems All normal body processes.

paracrine hormones Hormones that diffuse through intracellular spaces to their target.

pathophysiology The study of how normal physiological processes are altered by disease.

positive feedback A signal within a feedback loop that causes an action within that loop to increase.

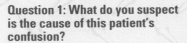

Case Study Answers

Question 1: What do you suspect is the cause of this patient's confusion?

Answer: Systemic hypothermia would be high on the list but you still need to suspect other causes of altered mental status, such as stroke, transient ischemic attack, head injury, diabetes, hypoxia, and seizure.

Question 2: What additional assessment or diagnostic tools should you consider using with this patient?

Answer: On the basis of the patient's cold skin and history of diabetes, it would be appropriate to obtain a tympanic temperature (because he might have a low body temperature) and obtain a few drops of blood for a determination of the patient's level of blood glucose (since he has a history of diabetes).

Question 3: What is the significance of the patient's uncontrollable shivering?

Answer: Shivering is a normal compensatory mechanism that the body uses to create heat. It is a good sign that the body is trying to bring its temperature back to the normal range. A lack of shivering might indicate that the hypothermia is so severe that his body's thermoregulatory mechanism has already failed.

Question 4: Which homeostatic mechanism has been affected by the prolonged exposure to the cold?

Answer: The homeostatic mechanism that has been affected is the body's thermometer, which is called thermoregulation. The body normally maintains its temperature at a steady 98.6°F, or 37.0°C. Thermoregulation has one of the major roles of the metabolic process. The body's metabolism generates body heat and requires fuel (food) to burn, just as a furnace needs fuel to heat. In addition to the exposure to cold, the patient had not eaten and thus had low fuel reserves.

Question 5: What are the potential causes of the patient's altered mental status?

Answer: The patient's glucose reading is low at 60 mg/dL. The normal range is 80 to 120 mg/dL. Low levels of blood glucose can cause confusion and unconsciousness, and, if not treated promptly, coma and death. There are many reasons that a patient can have an altered mental status. Consider causes such as head injury, seizure, stroke or transient ischemic attack, hypoxia, electrolyte imbalance, ECG abnormality, hypothermia or hyperthermia, an overdose of drugs or alcohol, and complications of diabetes. The patient's altered mental status in this case is most likely a combination of low blood glucose levels and hypothermia.

Question 6: Now that you have learned more about this patient's medical history, what do you suspect?

Answer: The cold outside temperature combined with the patient's history of diabetes and lack of eating a scheduled meal quickly exhausted his energy reserves and his ability to produce body heat. With the onset of confusion, the patient was unable to seek help and became colder and more confused.

Question 7: By observing the patient's response to the treatment provided, which condition, hypothermia or hypoglycemia (low blood glucose level), is quicker to reverse?

Answer: When the brain gets the sugar it needs through intake of food or IV, the body responds quickly. Raising the body's temperature is a slow process, and it must be accomplished slowly to prevent an adverse reaction. In the emergency department this can be done by warming up the core of the body with warm inhaled oxygen, warm IV fluids, specialty blankets, heating lamps, and more aggressive maneuvers such as heart-lung bypass and dialysis.

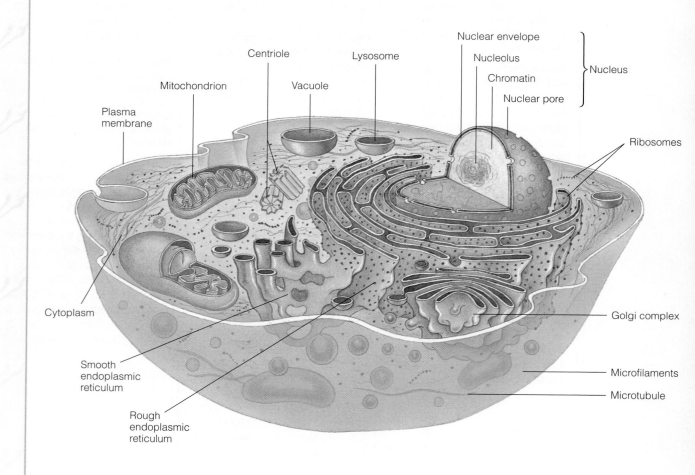

Centriole

Mitochondrion

Plasma
membrane

Vacuole

Lysosome

Nuclear envelope

Nucleolus

Chromatin

Nuclear pore

Nucleus

Ribosomes

Cytoplasm

Golgi complex

Smooth
endoplasmic
reticulum

Microfilaments

Microtubule

Rough
endoplasmic
reticulum

Cells and Tissues

OBJECTIVES

Cognitive

1-6.1 Discuss cellular adaptation. (p 21–23)

Additional Objectives*

1. List the major cellular organelles. (p 18)
2. Discuss the functions of the cellular organelles. (p 18)
3. Describe the four major tissue types. (p 19)
4. Define and give examples of atrophy, hypertrophy, hyperplasia, dysplasia, and metaplasia. (p 22–23)

*These are noncurriculum objectives.

www.Paramedic.EMSzone.com

TECHNOLOGY

Online Chapter Pretest

Vocabulary Explorer

Anatomy Review

Web Links

Chapter FEATURES

Case Studies

Physiology Tips

Medication Tips

Paramedic Safety Tips

Special Needs Tips

Vital Vocabulary

Prep Kit

Cells

Cells can be broken down into two general groups: nonspecialized and specialized. Cells become specialized through the process of __differentiation__, in which the cells mature and acquire the features of specialized cells. These specialized cells function or act in concert with similar cells to perform complex tasks within the body. Immature cells, called *stem cells,* are often able to differentiate into a variety of different cell types. Mature cells are also referred to as fully differentiated cells.

Cellular Components and Organelles

Nearly all cells, except red blood cells and platelets, have three main components: a nucleus, cytoplasm, and a cell membrane. The __nucleus__ contains the genetic material, called __chromatin__, and the __nucleoli__, which are rounded, dense structures that contain __ribonucleic acid (RNA)__. RNA is the substance in cells responsible for controlling cellular activities. The nucleus is surrounded by a membrane, called the __nuclear envelope__, and the nucleus itself is embedded in the __cytoplasm__. The cytoplasm

is a substance consisting of a combination of fluid and __organelles__. The organelles are tiny components of cells that are designed to carry out the processes necessary for life within each cell. Each cell is surrounded by a __cell membrane__. The major organelles include the following (▼ **Figure 2-1**):

- __Ribosomes__ – organelles that contain RNA and protein. They interact with RNA from other parts of the cell, joining amino acid chains together to form proteins.
- __Endoplasmic reticulum__ – a series of membranes in which fats (lipids) and very specific proteins are manufactured.
- __Golgi complex__ – a set of membranes within the cytoplasm associated with the formation of various carbohydrate (sugar) and complex protein molecules.
- __Lysosomes__ – membrane-bound vesicles that contain a variety of enzymes. These enzymes function as an intracellular digestive system.
- __Mitochondria__ – small, rod-like organelles that function as the metabolic center of the cell. The mitochondria produce __adenosine triphosphate (ATP)__, which is the major energy source for the body.

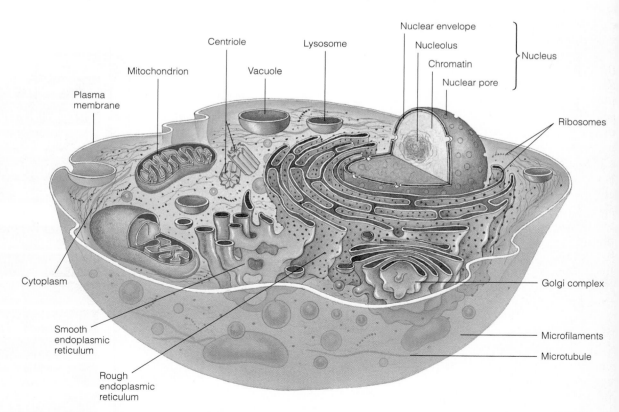

Figure 2-1 The structure of a cell. Note that the cell is divided into the nuclear and cytoplasmic compartments. The cytoplasm is packed with a variety of structures called the organelles, in which the cell carries out many functions.

Physiology Tip

Mitochondria contain a small set of chromosomes that are different from the genetic material in the nucleus. Abnormalities in mitochondrial chromosomes lead to a variety of mitochondrial disorders. The list of diseases associated with abnormalities in mitochondrial DNA is extensive. Both sudden infant death syndrome and some forms of hereditary cardiomyopathy occur as a result of mitochondrial chromosomal abnormalities.

Tissues

Tissues are composed of groups of similar cells working together for a common function. Anatomically, tissues are classified as one of the following four types: epithelial, connective, muscle, and nerve. Organs consist of various tissue types working together for a common purpose (eg, the heart contains muscle, nervous, and connective tissue). Organ systems consist of several organs working together for a common purpose (eg, the cardiovascular system consists of the heart, lungs, and blood vessels).

Epithelium is a type of tissue that covers all of the external surfaces of the body. Epithelial tissue also lines hollow organs within the body, such as the intestines, blood vessels, and bronchial tubes. In addition to providing a protective barrier, epithelial tissues function in the absorption of nutrients in the intestines and the secretion of various body substances. For example, the sweat glands in the dermis layer of the skin, specifically the stratified squamous epithelial cells, produce a solution containing urea and salt. Epithelium is broken down into specific types of cells that serve different functions. In addition to the ability of the stratified squamous epithelial cells to protect the underlying skin from sunlight, the simple columnar epithelium lines the small intestine and is designed to absorb nutrients from the foods we eat. Different types of epithelium are shown in ▶ Figure 2-2.

Epithelial cells that line the inside of blood vessels are termed endothelial cells. The endothelial lining of blood vessels (endothelium) performs several vital functions. It regulates the flow of blood through the vessel and also regulates clotting of the blood (coagulation).

Connective tissue binds the other types of tissue together. Extracellular matrix is a nonliving

Case Study

Case Study, Part 1

Your unit is dispatched to a hotel near the city's conference center for a 36-year-old man who has been electrocuted. After arriving, the general supervisor on the scene tells you that the patient was working on an electrical panel and was shocked when one of his tools made contact with the box. He advises you that the power has been shut off and directs you to the patient who has been moved from the area where the electrocution occurred. The patient is alert, sitting down, and has a severe burn on his left hand and arm.

Your general impression is that the patient is in moderate to severe distress due to the pain from the burn. As he describes what happened, it is clear that his airway and breathing are adequate. His distal pulse is fast and regular. You cut away his shirt and remove it completely to get a better look. Then you obtain a set of vital signs.

According to your local protocol, ALS is requested. This patient's priority is high and transport will begin as soon as you are prepared to transport. If the ALS unit is not yet on the scene, you can attempt to arrange an intercept en route to the hospital.

Initial Assessment

Recording time
0 minutes

Appearance
Moderate to severe distress due to pain

Level of consciousness
Alert and oriented to person, place, and day of the week

Airway
Open and clear

Vital Signs

Pulse rate/quality
110 beats/min, irregular, and strong

Blood pressure
154/90 mm Hg

Respiratory rate/depth
24 breaths/min, adequate

Question 1: Which tissues do you suspect may be affected in this patient's injury?

Question 2: From your findings on the initial assessment, which organ systems have been immediately affected?

Question 3: Although your patient's airway is intact, what are other important concerns with this electrical burn for you to consider?

Question 4: Why is ALS needed and what care might they provide for this patient?

CASE STUDY

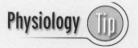

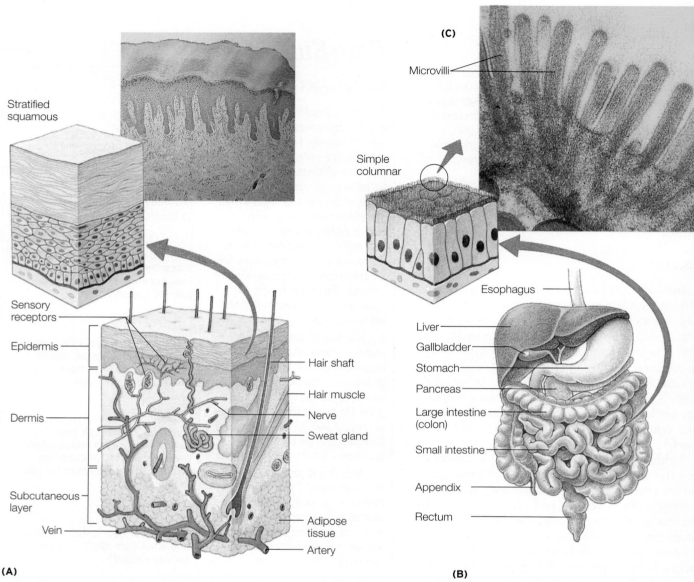

Figure 2-2 Different types of epithelial cells have different functions. **A.** A cross-section of skin showing the stratified squamous epithelium of the epidermis, which protects the underlying skin from sunlight. **B.** The simple columnar epithelium lining the small intestine is specialized for absorption. **C.** The folds or microvilli in the intestine increase the surface area for absorption.

Physiology Tip

Recent research has shown that dysfunction of the endothelium is at the root of atherosclerosis, heart failure, and shock.

substance consisting of protein fibers, nonfibrous protein, or fluid that separates connective tissue cells from one another. Collagen is the major protein comprising the extracellular matrix. There are at least 12 types of collagen, with types I, II, and III as the most abundant. Alterations in collagen structure resulting from abnormal genes or abnormal processing of collagen proteins results in numerous diseases (eg, scurvy). Bone and cartilage are subtypes of connective tissue. <u>Adipose tissue</u> is a special type of connective tissue that contains large amounts of lipids (fat).

<u>Muscle tissue</u> is located within the substance of the body and invariably enclosed by connective tissue. Muscle is characterized by its ability to contract. Muscles overlie the framework of the skeleton and are classified by both structure and function. Structurally, muscle tissue is either <u>striated</u>, in which microscopic bands or striations can be seen, or <u>nonstriated</u>, also called smooth. Functionally, muscle is either voluntary (consciously controlled) or involuntary (not normally under conscious control). The three types of muscle are <u>skeletal muscle</u> (striated voluntary), <u>cardiac muscle</u> (striated involuntary), and <u>smooth muscle</u> (nonstriated involuntary) (▶ Figure 2-3). Most of the muscles used voluntarily in day-to-day activities are skeletal muscles. The heart consists of cardiac muscle and has unique abilities to contract and generate impulses.

Smooth muscle lines most glands, digestive organs, lower airways, and vessels. When a patient's brain senses the need to respond to an environmental stimulus by vasoconstriction, the vessels in the periphery react. The smooth muscle in the bronchioles can vasoconstrict during an asthma attack, leading to wheezing and difficulty moving air out of the lungs. A bronchodilator is specifically designed to dilate the bronchioles during incidents of reactive airway disease, such as an asthma attack; this medication dilates the bronchioles and ultimately makes it easier for the patient to breathe. Smooth muscle is also responsible for constriction and dilation of the pupil of the eye when it is exposed to changes in light levels.

<u>Nerve tissue</u> includes the brain, spinal cord, and peripheral nerves. It is characterized by its ability to transmit nerve impulses. <u>Peripheral nerves</u> include all of the nerves that extend from the brain and spinal cord, exiting from between the vertebrae to various parts of the body. Neurons are the main conducting cells of nerve tissue. The cell body of the neuron includes the nucleus and is the site of most

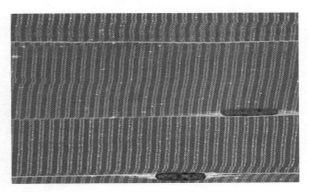

(A)

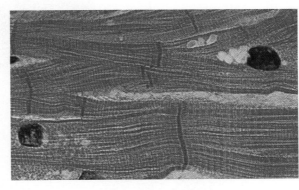

(B)

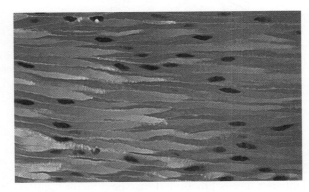

(C)

Figure 2-3 Light micrograph of the types of muscle tissue. A. Skeletal. B. Cardiac. C. Smooth.

cellular functions. <u>Dendrites</u> receive electrical impulses from the axons of other nerve cells and conduct them toward the cell body. <u>Axons</u> typically conduct electrical impulses away from the cell body. Each neuron has only one axon but may have several dendrites (▶ Figure 2-4).

Cell and Tissue Adaptations

When cells are exposed to adverse conditions, they go through a process of adaptation to protect themselves from injury. In some situations, the cells

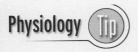

Physiology Tip

The suffix -*itis* means inflammation. The term <u>neuritis</u> refers to inflammation of a nerve. The suffix -*pathy* means disease of; thus, <u>neuropathy</u> is disease of a nerve. A complication of diabetes mellitus is diabetic neuropathy, which causes the patient to have abnormal sensations, particularly in the legs and feet.

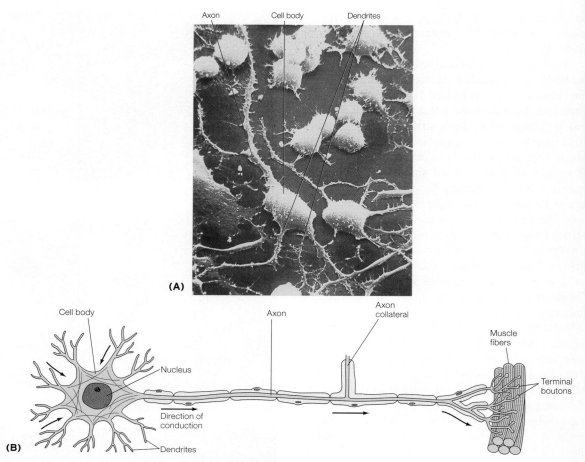

Figure 2-4 The neuron. **A.** A scanning electron micrograph of the cell body and dendrites of a multipolar neuron, which resides in the central nervous system. **B.** Collateral branches may occur along the length of the axon. When the axon terminates, it branches many times, ending on individual muscle fibers.

change permanently; in others, they change their structure and function temporarily. Although early stages of a successful adaptation response may enhance a cell's function, it may be difficult to differentiate pathological responses and an extreme adaptation. Examples of adaptations include atrophy, hypertrophy, hyperplasia, dysplasia, and metaplasia:

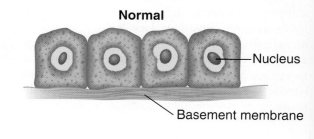

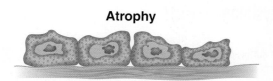

Figure 2-5 Atrophy—normal cells versus atrophied cells.

- <u>Atrophy</u> – a decrease in cell size leading to a decrease in the size of the tissue and organ. The actual number of cells remains unchanged; the cells decrease in size in order to cope with less-than-favorable conditions, or lack of use, for a period of time. The relationship between normal cells and atrophied cells is illustrated in ▶ **Figure 2-5**. This could easily occur as a result of a patient's extremity being immobilized in a cast for 6 weeks for treatment of a fracture.

Physiology Tip

An example of atrophy occurs in a leg that has been in a cast for 6 weeks or more. After the cast is removed, it is not uncommon for patients to find that the muscle has atrophied. For athletes, this is a serious problem that can cause a setback in their performance.

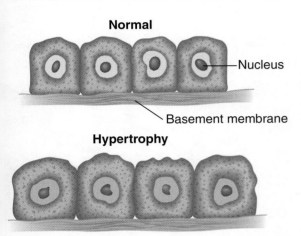

Normal

Nucleus

Basement membrane

Hypertrophy

Figure 2-6 Hypertrophy—normal cells versus hypertrophied cells.

- <u>Hypertrophy</u> – an increase in the size of the cells leading to an increase in tissue and organ size. An example of hypertrophy is the left ventricle of a patient who has diseased valves and arteries. The ventricle enlarges to compensate for a defect, such as high resistance pressures from hypertension (high blood pressure). The relationship between normal cells and hypertrophied cells is illustrated in ▲ **Figure 2-6**.
- <u>Hyperplasia</u> – an increase in the actual number of cells, often due to hormonal stimulation. This excess growth often occurs in tumors, which may be either malignant or benign. The relationship between normal tissue and hyperplastic tissue is illustrated in ▶ **Figure 2-7**. Benign prostatic hyperplasia is an increase in the number of prostate cells. This condition occurs commonly in men older than 50 years. It may be asymptomatic or it may result in urinary difficulty. Some experts believe that this disease may be a precursor to prostate cancer.
- <u>Dysplasia</u> – an alteration in the size and shape of cells as in a tumor. The relationship

Case Study

Case Study, Part 2

You discover that the patient was knocked to the ground as a result of the shock. He denies having any injury as a result of the fall, however, and your physical examination results also show no injuries. The patient's lung sounds are clear, with no apparent injury from any possible smoke inhalation. The focused physical exam reveals burn damage down to the bone on two fingers and the thumb, or third-degree (full-thickness) burn. The patient's arm has burn damage that involves the dermis, or a second-degree (partial-thickness) burn. The patient's SAMPLE history includes the following: He takes no prescription medication but has an allergy to penicillin. He took an over-the-counter allergy medication in the morning for sneezing and hay fever. You place him on a cardiac monitor and get an SpO_2 reading. You begin treatment by administering high-flow oxygen via a nonrebreathing mask and bandage and splint the injured hand and arm. Now you move the patient onto the stretcher and into the ambulance.

Focused Physical Assessment

Recording time
5 minutes

Lung sounds
Clear

Skin signs
Normal in the unaffected areas, second- and third-degree burns on the arm and hand

Diagnostic Tools

SpO_2
100%

Electrocardiogram
Sinus tachycardia at a rate of 110 beats/min, with premature unifocal ventricular contractions

Question 5: Will this type of injury cause cell and tissue adaptations?

Question 6: What is atrophy? Will the patient experience this through the healing process?

CASE STUDY

between normal cells and cells with dysplasia is illustrated in ▶ **Figure 2-8**. Dysplasia of epithelial cells can be the result of chronic inflammation or irritation (▶ **Figure 2-9**).

- <u>Metaplasia</u> – a cellular adaptation in which one cell changes to another type of cell (▶ **Figure 2-10**).

Normal

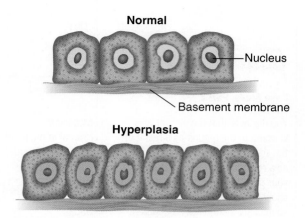

Nucleus

Basement membrane

Hyperplasia

Figure 2-7 Hyperplasia—normal tissue versus hyperplastic tissue.

Normal

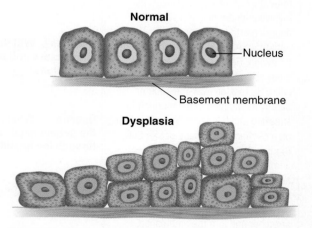

Nucleus

Basement membrane

Dysplasia

Figure 2-8 Dysplasia—normal tissue versus dysplastic tissue.

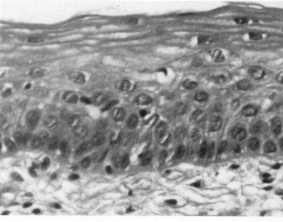

(A)

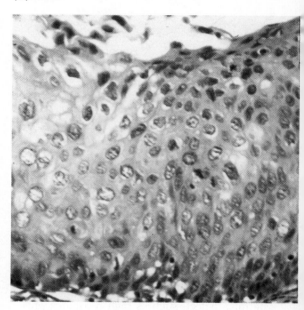

(B)

Figure 2-9 Nonkeratinized stratified squamous epithelium. A. With dysplastic epithelium. B. Note variation in nuclear size, polarity, and staining reaction (original magnification, ×400).

Physiology Tip

Changes in the lower esophagus from the normal squamous cell epithelium (flat, nonglandular) to columnar epithelium (columns, glandlike, more similar to stomach cells) result in Barrett's esophagitis. This lesion is a response to acid reflux and has a high incidence of progression to cancer of the esophagus. Not every disease or condition has a specific presentation that would be found by the paramedic in the field, considering the focused nature of a paramedic's assessment and the short duration that the patient is typically under the paramedic's care. Barrett's esophagitis could, however, present as chest pain (heartburn) or dysphagia (from a narrowing by the cancer).

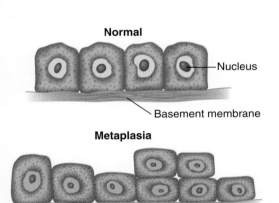

Normal

Nucleus

Basement membrane

Metaplasia

Figure 2-10 Metaplasia–normal tissue versus metaplastic tissue.

Case Study

Case Study, Part 3

Just as the patient has been moved to the ambulance the medic unit arrives on the scene. As transport is begun, the medic obtains IV access and you notify the hospital of the patient's condition and your ETA. Medical control authorizes the paramedic to use morphine relief of the patient's intense pain. En route you perform an ongoing assessment of the patient. The patient's vital signs are stable, and the morphine seems to be helping to reduce the pain from a 10/10 to a 5/10. The irregular heartbeat is improving. The patient is frightened and worried that he may have lost the use of his hand. You provide psychological support and try to answer his questions as truthfully as possible.

Ongoing Assessment

Recording time
20 minutes

Appearance
Moderate distress

Mental status
Worried and frightened

Vital Signs

Pulse rate/quality
96 beats/min, strong and more regular than before

Blood pressure
130/80 mm Hg

Respiratory rate/depth
20 breaths/min and adequate

SpO$_2$
100%

Electrocardiogram
Normal sinus rhythm at a rate of 96 beats/min, with occasional unifocal premature ventricular contractions

Question 7: What functional muscle type has been damaged in the hand and arm?

Question 8: The patient has a burn injury affecting the fatty part of the upper arm. Is fat a tissue, organ, or organ system? How is this soft-tissue injury managed in the field?

Case Study

Case Study, Part 4

Completion of the Case Study

While en route to the hospital, the medic administered additional morphine to help reduce the patient's severe pain. He has rough times ahead with the high risk of infection, multiple surgeries, healing, physical therapy, and more. The steps you have taken with him so far—keeping the wound clean, pain management, and psychological support—will make a significant difference in the outcome for this patient.

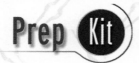

Chapter Summary

- Cells can be thought of in two general groupings of either specialized or nonspecialized. Specialized cells differentiate from nonspecialized stem cells during the cell maturation process.

- All cells except red blood cells and platelets have three main components: a nucleus, cytoplasm, and a cell membrane.

- The nucleus contains the genetic material and nucleoli—rounded, dense structures that contain ribonucleic acid (RNA), which is responsible for controlling cellular activities. The nucleus is embedded in the cytoplasm, a combination of fluid and organelles—components that carry out the processes necessary for life within each cell. The cell is surrounded by a cell membrane.

- There are four major tissue types. Epithelial tissue covers the internal and external surfaces of the body, including the linings of vessels. Connective tissue supports and binds other tissue types together. Muscle is characterized by its ability to contract. Nervous tissue is characterized by its ability to transmit nerve impulses.

- When cells are exposed to adverse conditions, they go through a process of adaptation to protect themselves from injury. In some situations, the cells change permanently; in others, they change their structure and function temporarily. Examples of adaptations include atrophy, hypertrophy, hyperplasia, dysplasia, and metaplasia.

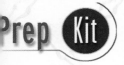

Vital Vocabulary

adenosine triphosphate (ATP) The major energy carrier molecule in the cell that is composed of ribose sugar, adenine, and three phosphate groups.

adipose tissue A connective tissue containing large amounts of lipids.

atrophy A decrease in cell size leading to a decrease in the size of the tissue and organ.

axons Part of the neuron that conducts the impulses away from the cell body.

cardiac muscle Striated involuntary muscle of the heart that contracts and generates impulses.

cell membrane The membrane surrounding the cell that is made up of fat and protein, which separates it from the other cells.

chromatin Long, threadlike fibers in the nucleus of the cell that contain DNA and proteins.

connective tissue Tissue that serves to bind various tissue types together.

cytoplasm A combination of fluid and organelles that comprises the contents of a cell exclusive of the nucleus.

dendrites Part of the neuron that receives impulses from the axon and contains vesicles for release of neurotransmittors.

differentiation Specialization of a stem cell into a mature cell with specialized features and function.

dysplasia An alteration in the size and shape of cells as in a tumor.

endoplasmic reticulum Cell organelles in which lipids and specific proteins are manufactured.

endothelial cells Specific types of epithelial cells that serve the function of lining the blood vessels.

epithelium Type of tissue that covers all external surfaces of the body.

Golgi complex Organelle characterized by a set of membranes, found within the cytoplasm, that are associated with the formation of carbohydrates and complex proteins.

hyperplasia An increase in the actual number of cells, often due to hormonal stimulation.

hypertrophy An increase in the size of the cells leading to an increase in tissue and organ size.

lysosomes Membrane-bound vesicles containing enzymes that act as part of the cell's digestive system.

metaplasia A cellular adaptation in which one cell changes to another type of cell.

mitochondria The metabolic center or powerhouse of the cell. They are small and rod-shaped organelles.

muscle tissue Specialized tissue designed to contract.

nerve tissue The tissue responsible for transmitting impulses throughout the body. Nerve tissue is found in the brain, spinal cord, and peripheral nerves.

neuritis An inflammation of the nerves.

neuropathy A disease of the nerves that often causes abnormal sensations. Often found in advanced stages of diabetes.

nonstriated A type of muscle tissue that is smooth and does not have visible bands.

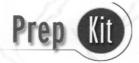

nuclear envelope The membrane surrounding the nucleus of a cell.

nucleoli Structures in the nuclei of a cell that exist temporarily during interphase. Regions of DNA that are active in the production of RNA are also referred to as nucleoli.

nucleus A cellular organelle that contains the genetic information. The nucleus controls the function and structure of a cell.

organs A series of various tissue types working together to accomplish a common function.

organelles Internal cellular structures that carry out specific functions for the cell.

organ systems Several organs working together for a common purpose.

peripheral nerves All of the nerves of the body extending from the brain and spinal cord.

ribonucleic acid (RNA) Nucleic acid associated with controlling cellular activities.

ribosomes Organelles that contain RNA and proteins.

skeletal muscle Striated voluntary muscle found in the body.

smooth muscle Nonstriated involuntary muscle that is responsible for constriction and dilation of the pupils as well as lining the glands, digestive organs, lower airway, and vessels.

striated Another name for skeletal muscle tissue, containing bands of fibers that can be seen under a microscope.

tissues Groups of cells working together for a common function such as the epithelial tissue to cover the outermost surfaces of the body.

Case Study Answers

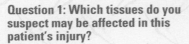

Question 1: Which tissues do you suspect may be affected in this patient's injury?

Answer: Tissues are groups of similar cells working together for a common function. A body organ is composed of various tissue types working together for a common purpose. An organ system consists of several organs working together for a common purpose. The tissues that would be affected include the epithelial tissues, which cover surfaces of the body. There may also be damage to the nervous tissue and the heart muscle tissue from the current.

Question 2: From your findings on the initial assessment, which organ systems have been immediately affected?

Answer: The burn has directly affected the skin or integumentary system, underlying muscles, and the cardiovascular system (irregular heart beat).

Question 3: Although your patient's airway is intact, what are other important concerns with this electrical burn for you to consider?

Answer: The depth of the burn on the hand and arm will determine which tissue types have been affected. If the burn is circumferential, it is very serious because the pressures in the tissue can build up, and a tourniquet may develop in the patient's extremity. Because the patient was burned with electricity, the current had to enter and exit his body. The entry point is somewhat obvious in the hand but the exit point is not as obvious. Try to find it when you perform the physical examination.

Question 4: Why is ALS needed and what care might they provide for this patient?

Answer: ALS care is needed because of the type of burn. The full extent of an electrical burn is not always clear in the field. The pathway of the current traveling through the patient's body may have crossed the heart, potentially disrupting the normal conduction system of the heart. ALS will provide resuscitative care, including fluid resuscitation, monitoring the patient for dysrhythmias, and pain management.

Question 5: Will this type of injury cause cell and tissue adaptations?

Answer: Yes, a severe burn injury is one example of how cells and tissue will permanently change their structure and function. Severe scarring and damage to muscle and connective tissues usually leaves the patient with limited function in an extremity. Nerve tissue damage is often permanent as well and may limit the range of motion in the future.

Question 6: What is atrophy? Will the patient experience this through the healing process?

Answer: Atrophy is the decrease in the cell size of the tissue and organ, which occurs with inactivity or decreased use. This patient, in addition to the tissue damage from the burn, will experience atrophy in some muscles due to the limited use of his arm during the healing process.

Question 7: What functional muscle type has been damaged in the hand and arm?

Answer: The muscles of the hand and arm are primarily voluntary skeletal muscle and they may be permanently damaged by the burn. It is also possible that some damage can occur to involuntary smooth muscle in the walls of the vessels within the hand and arm.

Question 8: The patient has a burn injury affecting the fatty part of the upper arm. Is fat a tissue, organ, or organ system? How is this soft-tissue injury managed in the field?

Answer: Fat is a special kind of connective tissue that contains large amounts of lipids (fats). You will need to cover the burned area with a dry sterile dressing and bandage. Be sure to remove the patient's jewelry because the extremity will begin to swell. The patient should receive an IV line and fluid resuscitation. It is not appropriate to start the IV in the injured arm unless absolutely necessary.

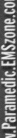

CASE STUDY ANSWERS

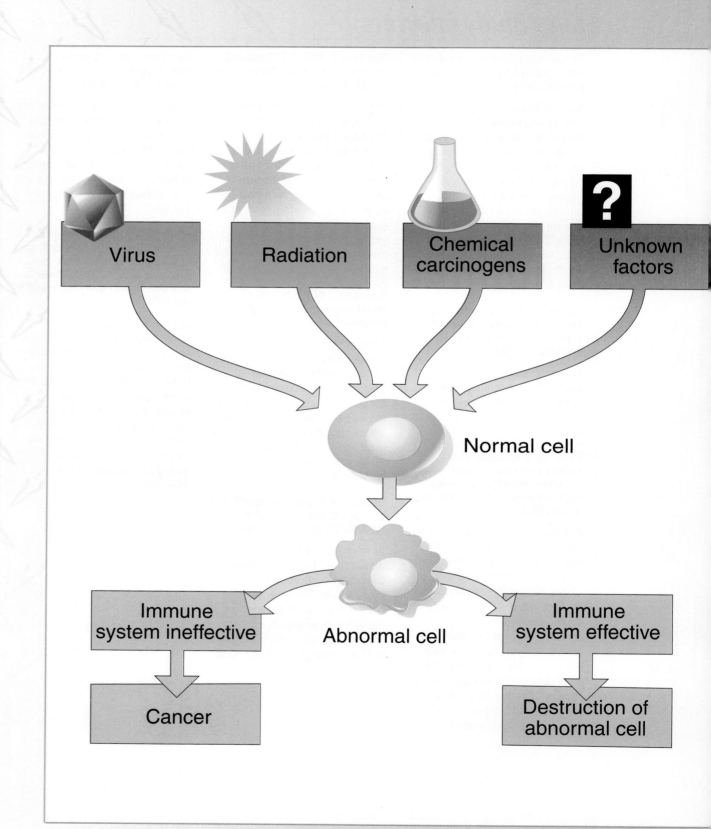

Cell and Tissue Injury

3

OBJECTIVES

Cognitive

-6.2 Describe cellular injury and cellular death. (p 32)

-6.3 Describe the factors that precipitate disease in the human body. (p 36)

-6.28 Describe the systemic manifestations that result from cellular injury. (p 32)

Additional Objectives*

1. List the manifestations of cellular death. (p 32)
2. Compare and contrast necrosis and apoptosis. (p 33)
3. Describe the role of free radicals in hypoxic injury. (p 35)

*These are noncurriculum objectives.

Chapter TECHNOLOGY

www.Paramedic.EMSzone.com

- Online Chapter Pretest
- Vocabulary Explorer
- Anatomy Review
- Web Links

Chapter FEATURES

- Case Studies
- Physiology Tips
- Medication Tips
- Paramedic Safety Tips
- Special Needs Tips
- Vital Vocabulary
- Prep Kit

Cell Injury

Cellular injury may result from various causes, such as hypoxia (the most common cause), chemical injury, infectious injury, immunologic injury, mechanical injury, and inflammatory injury. The manifestations of cell injury and death depend on how many and which types of cells are injured.

Manifestations of Cellular Injury and Death

Manifestations of cellular injury occur at the microscopic (structural) and functional levels. Common microscopic abnormalities as seen in the cardiac cell undergoing necrosis from hypoxemia for an extended period of time (▶ **Figure 3-1**) include:

- Cell swelling
- Rupture of cell membranes
- Rupture of nuclear membranes
- Breakdown of nuclear material (chromosomes)

This damage often results in a change in cell shape and its function.

Functional changes may include:

- Inability to use oxygen appropriately
- Development of intracellular acidosis
- Accumulation of toxic waste products
- Inability to metabolize nutrients

Damage to and functional changes in individual cells often have an impact on the entire organism. The degree of systemic involvement depends on exactly which individual cells are injured, as well as the extent of the injury. In some cases only minor systemic abnormalities are noted, such as fever.

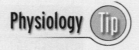

Physiology Tip

Alterations in function become apparent early. Structural changes occur later, and are usually noted only after critical biochemical damage has already occurred (eg, brain atrophy after an anoxic injury). Anoxic injury that is secondary to a prolonged period of hypoxia (ie, from prolonged cardiac arrest with a return of spontaneous circulation) results in immediate coma and loss of function. Structural changes seen on CT can take much longer to develop.

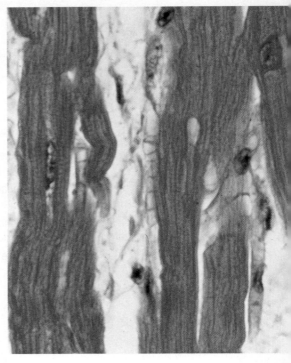

(A)

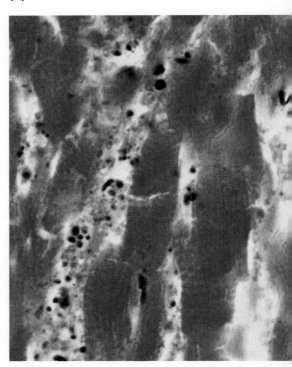

(B)

Figure 3-1 Comparison of cardiac muscle fibers. **A.** With necrotic fibers. **B.** Note fragmentation of fibers, loss of nuclear staining, and fragmented bits of nuclear debris. When the cell injured it swells, resulting in nuclear membrane rupture and breakdown of the nuclear material leaking the cell's contents (original magnification, ×400).

Other times, entire organ systems fail and the patient's situation becomes critical (eg, kidney failure). Four intracellular systems are particularly vulnerable to injury:

1. Aerobic respiration – mitochondrial oxidative phosphorylation and the production of adenosine triphosphate (ATP).
2. Integrity of cell membranes – the ionic and osmotic homeostasis of the cell depends on proper function of the cell membrane. Regardless of cause, virtually all cell injury results in damage to cell membranes.
3. Protein synthesis.
4. Genetic apparatus of the cell.

All body systems are connected in some manner. Dysfunction in one system inevitably affects other systems. When the homeostatic balance in the body is upset, the "scales" can shift in an unfavorable direction.

Cell injury may, up to a point, be reversible with proper treatment. Irreversible injury occurs once cells have passed a "point of no return," after which no treatment will help. Cell death is followed by **necrosis**, a process by which the cell breaks down. The cell membrane becomes abnormally permeable, leading to the influx of electrolytes and fluids. The cell swells, along with its organelles. Lysosomes (► **Figure 3-2**) release enzymes that destroy intracellular components. These processes occur during and after actual cell death.

Apoptosis is normal, genetically programmed cell death. During apoptosis, cells exhibit characteristic nuclear changes. Typically, cells die in well-defined clusters rather than in a random fashion. The molecular mechanism of cell death involves the activation of genes that code for proteins known as **caspases**. You can think of these proteins as cellular "cyanide," because their production essentially leads to cell suicide. Unlike death from disease processes, proteins and DNA undergo controlled degradation instead of necrosis that allows them to be taken up and reused by neighboring cells. The necrosis is not generally a cause of death, rather a result of death. Apoptosis thus allows the body to eliminate a cell but still "recycle" many of its components. Pathologically, there is a characteristic *lack* of inflammation in areas that have undergone apoptotic death. This is strikingly different, for example, from cells that have undergone necrosis from hypoxia or cellular toxins; in these situations, an inflammatory response is typical.

Apoptosis is unique in that it is genetically programmed into the cell as a part of normal development, organogenesis, immune function, and tissue

Case Study

Case Study, Part 1

Your unit has been dispatched to the site of an industrial accident with entrapment. The fire department and special operations rescue team are on the scene when you arrive and fill you in on the situation. There is a 28-year-old conscious man whose legs are trapped under a slab of concrete. He was working in the building when a truck drove into the building, collapsing a wall and the upper floor onto him. The driver of the truck is being treated by another EMS crew.

The structure had to be stabilized before you could gain access to the patient, which took almost 40 minutes. Now your general impression of the patient is that he is alert and anxious. He is able to speak clearly as he tells you that the pain in his legs is very bad. His breathing is nonlabored through the oxygen mask that a rescuer placed on him. His skin is warm and moist, and the distal pulses in his arms are strong, fast, and regular. His legs are not yet accessible.

The rescue team tells you that they are waiting for low-pressure air bags and additional shoring materials to arrive before they can free the patient. You let the patient know what is happening with the rescue and obtain a set of baseline vital signs. You also begin to ask about his medical history.

Initial Assessment

Recording time
40 minutes

Appearance
Conscious adult male whose legs are trapped under a slab of concrete

Level of consciousness
Alert and anxious

Airway
Open and able to speak

Vital Signs

Pulse rate/quality
118 beats/min, regular, strong

Blood pressure
126/78 mm Hg

Respiratory rate/depth
20 breaths/min, nonlabored

Question 1: Describe the initial progression of cell damage due to a crush injury.

Question 2: What might happen to the cells if the entrapment is prolonged for several hours?

Question 3: When cells become hypoxic, various compounds accumulate as a result of local inflammation. What are the earliest compounds produced as a response to this hypoxia and why are they the most dangerous?

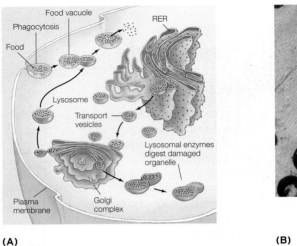

(A)

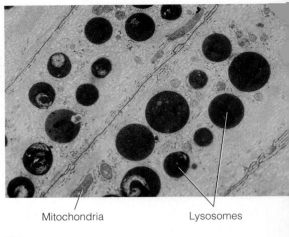

Mitochondria   Lysosomes

(B)

Figure 3-2 Lysosomes. **A.** The digestive enzymes of the lysosome are produced on the rough endoplasmic reticulum and transported to the Golgi complex for repackaging. Lysosomes produced by the Golgi complex fuse with food vacuoles; this allows their enzymes to mix with the contents of the food vacuole. The enzymes digest the contents, which diffuse through the membrane into the cytoplasm, where they are used. The membrane surrounding the lysosome helps protect the cell from digestive enzymes. **B.** An electron micrograph of lysosomes within a macrophage. The dark-staining bodies are the lysosomes, filled with digestive enzymes that are used by these cells to break down ingested material.

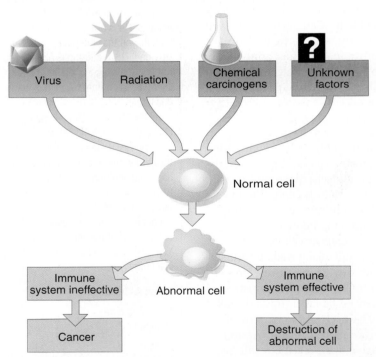

Figure 3-3 The onset of cancer. Viruses and other factors induce a normal cell to become abnormal. When the immune system is effective, it destroys abnormal cells, and no cancer develops. However, when abnormal cells evade the immune system, they form a tumor and then may become a spreading cancer.

growth. Apoptosis plays a normal role in aging, early development, menses, lactating breast tissue, thymus involution, and red blood cell turnover. It can also be activated prematurely by pathologic factors such as cell injury.

Premature stimulation of apoptosis results in early cell death, which occurs in some forms of heart failure. Another example of pathologic apoptosis is the death of hepatocytes (liver cells) in patients with viral hepatitis. The dying cells form lumps of chromatin known as *Councilman's bodies.* Factors that inhibit the normal course of apoptosis result in unwanted cellular proliferation. Examples include cancer and rheumatoid arthritis (uncontrolled synovial tissue proliferation). The process by which cancerous cells can develop from normal cells is illustrated in ◄ Figure 3-3.

Hypoxic Injury

Hypoxic injury is a common cause of cellular injury. It is also often deadly and may result from:

- Decreased amounts of oxygen in the air (eg, carbon monoxide poisoning).
- Loss of hemoglobin function (eg, carbon monoxide poisoning).
- Decreased number of red blood cells (eg, bleeding).
- Disease of the respiratory or cardiovascular system (eg, chronic obstructive pulmonary disease).
- Loss of cytochromes (mitochondrial proteins that convert oxygen to ATP; eg, cyanide poisoning).

Hypoxia alone is deleterious to cells; however, the damage does not stop there. Cells that are hypoxic for more than a few seconds produce **mediators** (substances) that often cause additional damage at local or distant body locations. The result is a vicious positive feedback cycle in which mediators lead to more cell damage, which leads to more hypoxia, then to further mediator production, and so forth.

The earliest and most dangerous mediators produced by cells in response to hypoxia are **free radicals**. These are molecules that are missing one electron in their outer shell. The presence of an odd, unpaired electron results in chemical instability (▼ Figure 3-4). Free radicals randomly attack cells and membranes in an attempt to "steal back" the missing

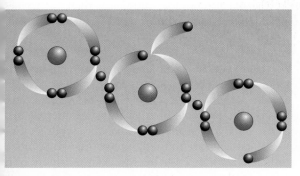

Figure 3-4 Free radicals are molecules that are missing one electron in their outside orbit. The presence of an odd, unpaired electron results in chemical instability. Each black dot represents an electron in the outer shell.

Case Study

Case Study, Part 2

The patient tells you that he has a history of seizures and takes Dilantin (phenytoin). He is allergic to Cipro (ciprofloxacin, an antibiotic). He is a smoker and asks if you can let him have a cigarette. You begin a focused physical exam and find that his lung sounds are clear. He has no pain on palpation of his head, neck, chest, and back. There are a few small abrasions on his hands and arms. At this point his injuries are limited to the crushed lower extremities. You know, however, that this type of injury can affect other body systems and disrupt the patient's homeostasis. The sudden release of pressure on his legs will cause a release of harmful substances into his bloodstream. He will need IV fluids, and consideration should be given to addressing the acidosis and hyperkalemia. You attach a pulse oximeter and obtain an ECG.

Focused Physical Assessment

Recording time
45 minutes

Appearance
No apparent injury or pain on palpation of his head, neck, chest, and back. Minor abrasions on the upper extremities.

Lung sounds
Clear

Diagnostic Tools

SpO_2
100%

Electrocardiogram
Sinus tachycardia at a rate of 120 beats/min with no ventricular ectopy

Question 4: What happens to a cell when it is damaged?

Question 5: What will happen to the cells when the concrete slab is lifted off the patient's legs? Is there any way to prepare for this reaction in the field?

Medication Tip

A goal in the management of the patient with a severe crush injury is alkalinization of the urine. To maintain the urine at a pH greater than 6.5, sodium bicarbonate, 50 mEq, is added to the initial IV fluids. This helps to control hyperkalemia and acidosis to prevent myoglobinuria renal failure. Alkalinization of the urine may be started in the field if the paramedic is given a direct medical order from medical control.

electron. The result is widespread and potentially deadly tissue damage.

Chemical Injury

Several chemicals injure and ultimately destroy cells. Examples of chemical agents that cause cellular injury include poisons, lead, carbon monoxide, ethanol, and pharmacologic agents.

- Poisons – Common poisons include cyanide and pesticides. Cyanide produces cell hypoxia by blocking oxidative phosphorylation in the mitochondria and preventing the metabolism of oxygen. Pesticides block an enzyme, acetyl-cholinesterase, thus preventing proper transmission of nerve impulses.

- Lead – Chronic ingestion of lead, such as that caused by chewing on windowsills painted with lead-based paint, leads to brain injury and neurologic dysfunction. There are several different mechanisms by which lead probably causes brain injury and neurologic dysfunction. Although all of lead's toxic effects cannot be tied together by a single unifying mechanism, its ability to substitute for calcium in the body (molecules of lead and calcium are a similar size) is a common factor in many of its toxic actions. It is likely that lead is "mistaken" for calcium in vital biochemical reactions, leading to abnormal results and dysfunction.

- Carbon monoxide – Carbon monoxide binds to hemoglobin, preventing adequate oxygenation of the tissues. Low levels cause nausea, vomiting, and headache. Higher levels result in death.

- Ethanol – In lower doses, ethanol causes the well-known effects of inebriation; higher doses result in severe central nervous depression, hypoventilation, and cardiovascular collapse.

- Pharmacologic agents – Some drugs produce toxic products when they are metabolized in the body, especially in "overdose conditions." Acetaminophen (Tylenol), in doses of more than 7.5 g/dL in an adult results in the accumulation of toxic intermediates that poison the liver and may lead to death.

Infectious Injury

Infectious injury to cells is caused by an invasion of either bacteria or viruses. **Virulence** measures the disease-causing ability of a microorganism. The pathogenicity of these microorganisms is a function of their ability to reproduce and cause disease within the human body. Bacteria may cause injury either by direct action on cells or by the production of toxins.

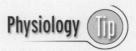

Physiology Tip

Chemical carcinogens, or cancer-causing agents, can be found everywhere in our environment. The exposure of workers to various chemicals used in industry can lead to cancer. Examples include:

- Naphthylamine found in dyes can cause bladder cancer.
- Nickel ore miners have a high rate of nasal cancer from breathing in nickel.
- Asbestos (previously used in insulation) can cause lung cancer.
- Arsenic in insecticides can lead to skin and lung cancer.
- Tar and nicotine from tobacco and cigarette smoke are leading causes of lung cancer.

Viruses often initiate an inflammatory response that leads to cell damage and patient symptoms.

The growth and survival of bacteria in the body depends on the effectiveness of the body's own defense mechanisms and the bacteria's ability to resist those mechanisms. The immune system helps to fight off foreign matter that the body perceives as harmful. A depressed immune system is present in many people: newborn infants, elderly patients, diabetics, and people with cancer or other chronic diseases.

Many bacteria have a capsule that protects them from ingestion and destruction by **phagocytes**—a kind of cell, including white blood cells, that engulfs and consumes foreign material such as microorganisms and debris (▶ **Figure 3-5**). Not all bacteria are encapsulated. *Mycobacterium tuberculosis* lacks a capsule, yet resists destruction. It can be transported by phagocytes throughout the body.

Bacteria also produce substances such as enzymes or toxins that can injure or destroy cells. These substances are usually referred to as either **exotoxins** or **endotoxins**. Staphylococci, streptococci, and *Clostridium tetani* secrete exotoxins into the medium surrounding the cell. Endotoxins are lipopolysaccharides that are part of the cell wall of Gram-negative bacteria. When large amounts of endotoxins are present in a patient's body, he or she may experience septic shock.

When cells are injured, circulating white blood cells are attracted to the site. White blood cells release endogenous **pyrogens** that cause a fever to develop. The body's most common reaction to the presence of bacteria is inflammation. Some bacteria have the ability to produce hypersensitivity

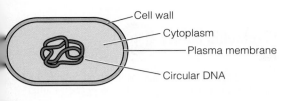

(A)

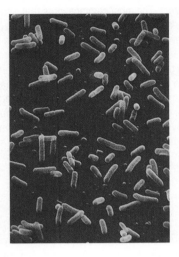

(B)

Figure 3-5 General structure of a bacterium. **A.** Bacteria come in many shapes and sizes, but all have a circular strand of DNA, cytoplasm, and a plasma membrane. Surrounding the membrane of many bacteria is a cell wall. **B.** An electron micrograph of salmonella bacteria. Many bacteria have a capsule that protects them from ingestion and destruction by phagocytes.

Physiology Tip

Fever is actually a feedback loop. Pyrogens produced by the invading organism and the body's own white blood cells cause the brain's hypothalamic thermoregulatory center to reset the body temperature at a higher level. This reset signals a constriction of the blood vessels that causes shivering, which in turn produces body heat and the measurable fever. The reason the patient feels cold and has the chills, even with the fever present, is that the body feels cold relative to the higher "set point." The body's higher core temperature is designed to both kill the microorganisms and stimulate the immune system to "attack." Once the invading microorganisms have been killed, the pyrogen level drops and the body returns the temperature to normal by dilating the blood vessels, sweating profusely, and allowing evaporation of the sweat to cool the body.

Case Study

Case Study, Part 3

At the scene you made direct contact with medical control and obtained orders to run in IV fluids and administer sodium bicarbonate. You also have an order for morphine for pain that is to be administered prior to lifting the concrete from the patient. All of your equipment is ready to go and you are prepared for the patient to experience acute shock or even cardiac arrest after he is freed. Throughout your care you have provided emotional and psychological support for the patient. The rescue team is ready, and so is the patient.

One hour and forty minutes into the rescue, the slab is lifted. The patient is secured on a long backboard and quickly moved to the ambulance so transport can begin. You remove the patient's shoes and socks and cut away the pants. His lower legs are severely crushed and he has no distal pulse in the right leg. You perform an ongoing assessment and update the emergency department on the patient's status while en route.

Ongoing Assessment

Recording time
1 hour 45 minutes

Mental status
Alert

Symptoms
Pain and paresthesia (pins and needles) in the left leg
No sensation in the right lower leg

Signs
Skin is pale, cool, and moist.
Severe tissue, muscle, and bone damage to the lower legs

Vital Signs

Pulse rate/quality
130 beats/min, regular and weak

Blood pressure
100/50 mm Hg

Respiratory rate/depth
28 breaths/min, slightly labored

Diagnostic Tools

SpO₂
SpO_2
100%

Electrocardiogram
Sinus tachycardia at 130 beats/min

Question 6: How does natural or normal cell death occur and what is it called?

Question 7: What is the major difference between normal cell death and cell death due to hypoxia or other injury?

CASE STUDY

Medication Tip

Since pyrogens act by affecting the hypothalamic thermoregulatory center, fever-reducing drugs, such as aspirin or acetaminophen, are designed to blunt the hypothalamic response. Antipyretics inhibit the production of prostaglandins, which stimulate the hypothalamus, causing fever. By blocking these, antipyretics blunt the hypothalamic response.

Paramedic Safety Tip

A significant exposure occurs when blood or body fluids come into contact with broken skin, the eyes, or other mucous membranes or through a parenteral (needle stick) contact. The most common virus that paramedics come into contact with in the field is hepatitis B, with 70,000 new infections reported annually in the United States. It is estimated that 500,000 Americans are currently infected with hepatitis, which causes inflammation of the liver. Always take body substance isolation precautions with all patients and have your personal protective equipment with you at all times. You should also always follow your agency's exposure control plan for the proper disposal of sharps.

reactions. The proliferation of microorganisms in the blood is called bacteremia, or sepsis.

Viral diseases are among the most common afflictions seen in humans. Viruses are intracellular parasites that take over the metabolic processes of the host cell and use the cell to help them replicate.

The protein coat that encapsulates most viruses protects them from phagocytosis. The replication of a virus occurs inside the host cell because viruses do not contain any of their own organelles. Viral infection of a host cell leads to a decreased synthesis of macromolecules that are vital to the host cell (▶ Figure 3-6). As opposed to bacteria, viruses do not produce exotoxins or endotoxins.

There may be a **symbiotic relationship** between a virus and normal cells that results in a persistent unapparent infection. Viruses have been known to evoke a strong immune response and can rapidly produce an irreversible, lethal injury in highly susceptible cells, as is the case with acquired immunodeficiency syndrome (AIDS).

Immunologic and Inflammatory Injury

Inflammation is a protective response that can occur without bacterial invasion. Infection is the invasion of microorganisms that causes cell or tissue injury, which leads to the inflammatory response. The immune system provides protection for the body by providing defenses to attack and removing foreign organisms such as bacteria or viruses.

The cellular membranes may be injured by direct contact with the cellular and chemical components of the immune or inflammatory process such as phagocytes (lymphocytes and macrophages), histamine, antibodies, and lymphokines. When cell membranes are altered, potassium leaks out of the cells and water flows inward. The result is swelling of the cell. The nuclear envelope, organelle membranes, and the cell membrane may all rupture, leading to death of the cell. The degree of swelling and membrane rupture depends on the severity of the immune and inflammatory response.

Other Injurious Factors

Genetic factors, nutritional imbalances, and physical agents can also cause cell injury and death. Examples of injurious genetic factors affecting cells include chromosomal disorders (eg, Down syndrome), premature development of atherosclerosis, and obesity (some cases). There are two ways an abnormal gene may develop in an individual: (1) by mutation of the gene during meiosis, which affects the newly formed fetus, or (2) by heredity. In trisomy 21 (Down syndrome), the child is born with an extra chromosome, usually number 21.

Good nutrition is required to maintain good health and assist the cells in fighting off disease. Examples of nutritional disorders that can injure cells and the organism as a whole include obesity, malnutrition, vitamin excess or deficiency, and mineral excess or deficiency. Any of these conditions can lead to alterations in physical growth, mental and intellectual retardation, and even death in some circumstances.

Physical agents, such as heat, cold, and radiation, may cause cell injury. Examples include burns, frostbite, radiation sickness, and tumors. The degree of cell injury that results is determined by both the strength of the agent and the length of exposure.

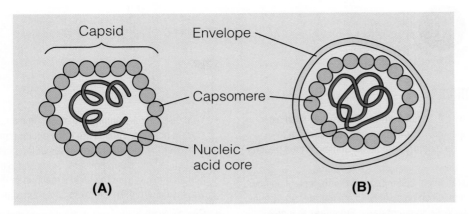

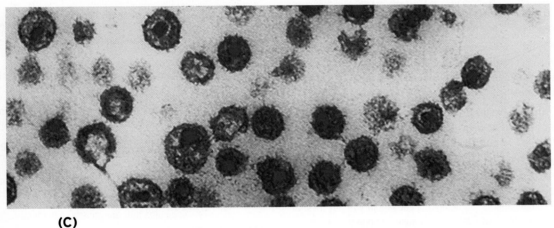

(C)

Figure 3-6 General structure of a virus. **A.** The virus consists of a nucleic acid core of either RNA or DNA. Surrounding the viral core is a layer of protein known as the capsid. Each protein molecule in the capsid is known as a capsomere. **B.** Some viruses have an additional protective coat known as the envelope. **C.** An electron micrograph of the human immunodeficiency virus (HIV).

Physiology Tip

Inflammation is a common response to many different stimuli, including infection, immune responses, and trauma.

Case Study

Case Study, Part 4

Completion of the Case Study

Transport to the trauma center was brief. En route the patient received more IV fluids and sodium bicarbonate. He exhibited signs and symptoms of shock but did not have any dysrhythmias. Your goal with this type of injury is to prevent sudden death and renal failure and salvage the lower limbs. The early treatment in the field to alkalize the urine with fluid and sodium bicarbonate was valuable. During the next 24 hours, he will continue to receive IV fluids and medication to maintain urine output. Maintaining urine output treats hypovolemia, keeps the kidneys functioning, corrects the acidosis, and treats the hyperkalemia (high potassium levels). This prevents cardiac dysrhythmias and renal failure. Your role in properly assessing this patient, involving medical direction, aggressive fluid resuscitation, and closely monitoring the patient, has been essential to his future recovery.

CASE STUDY

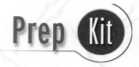

Chapter Summary

- Cellular injury can result from various causes, such as: chemical exposure, infectious agents, immunologic responses, inflammatory responses, and prolonged periods of hypoxia.

- The manifestations of cell injury and death depend on how many cells and which types of cells are injured. Alterations in function become apparent early. Structural changes occur later and are usually noted only after critical biochemical damage has already occurred.

- The most common microscopic abnormality observed is swelling of the cell and rupture of cell membranes. Release of enzymes from ruptured lysosomes often leads to cell death.

- Hypoxic injury may result from numerous causes. Hypoxia leads to the formation of free radicals, unstable molecules that often cause further injury.

- Several chemicals injure and ultimately destroy cells. Examples of chemical agents that cause cellular injury include poisons, lead, carbon monoxide, ethanol, and pharmacologic agents. Some agents cause injury at any level of ingestion (eg, cyanide); others cause damage when excessive amounts are ingested ("overdose conditions").

- Infectious injury to cells is caused by an invasion of either bacteria or viruses. Virulence measures the disease-causing ability of a microorganism. The pathogenicity of these microorganisms is a function of their ability to cause disease within the human body.

- Many bacteria have a capsule that protects them from ingestion and destruction by phagocytes—cells such as white blood cells, which engulf and consume foreign material such as microorganisms and debris. Not all bacteria are encapsulated. Bacteria also produce substances such as enzymes or toxins that can injure or destroy cells. These are usually referred to as either exotoxins or endotoxins.

- Viral diseases are among the most common afflictions seen in humans. Viruses are intracellular parasites that take over the metabolic processes of the host cell and use the cell to help them replicate. Signs and symptoms of viral infection result from the body's reaction to the virus. Viruses do not make exotoxins or endotoxins.

- Genetic factors, nutritional imbalances, and physical agents can also cause cell injury and death.

Vital Vocabulary

<u>apoptosis</u> The normal, genetically programmed death of a cell.

<u>caspases</u> Proteins whose production essentially leads to cell suicide.

<u>endotoxins</u> A metabolic poison produced chiefly by Gram-negative bacteria.

<u>exotoxins</u> A metabolic poison produced chiefly by Gram-positive bacteria.

<u>free radicals</u> Molecules that are missing one electron in their outer shells.

<u>mediators</u> Substances involved in the hypoxic injury process that cause additional local or remote injury when released.

<u>necrosis</u> A process by which the cell breaks down.

<u>phagocytes</u> Cells that engulf and consume foreign material such as microorganisms and debris.

<u>pyrogens</u> Microorganisms that affect the hypothalamic thermoregulatory center causing fever to occur.

<u>symbiotic relationship</u> An interrelationship between two populations of organisms in which there is a close and permanent association for mutual benefit.

<u>virulence</u> The disease-causing ability of a microorganism.

Case Study Answers

Question 1: Describe the initial progression of cell damage due to a crush injury.

Answer: The trauma directly to the soft tissue causes edema (swelling) and ischemia (tissue anemia). The cells in the crushed tissue are starved for oxygen and anaerobic metabolism occurs.

Question 2: What might happen to the cells if the entrapment is prolonged for several hours?

Answer: The progressing edema within the soft tissues causes the pressure to increase inside the muscle cells. A prolonged period of ischemia, greater than 6 to 8 hours, leads to tissue hypoxia (oxygen deprivation) and anoxia (permanent damage), and ultimately cell death.

Question 3: When cells become hypoxic, various compounds accumulate as a result of local inflammation. What are the earliest compounds produced as a response to this hypoxia and why are they the most dangerous?

Answer: In response to hypoxia, cells produce free radicals. They are highly reactive chemical intermediates that react with cell membranes, damaging them and leading to additional tissue damage.

Question 4: What happens to a cell when it is damaged?

Answer: Almost all cell damage results in damage to the cell wall. As the membranes weaken, they become abnormally permeable, and an influx of electrolytes (eg, calcium) and fluids causes swelling of the cell. Enzymes (eg, xanthine oxidase) are activated, leading to the formation of more toxic mediators (eg, uric acid).

Question 5: What will happen to the cells when the concrete slab is lifted off the patient's legs? Is there any way to prepare for this reaction in the field?

Answer: Many of the compounds described in the answer to question 4 will be released into the patient's systemic circulation. The result is often acute shock and cardiac arrest. In some EMS systems, the medical control physician may order an IV infusion as well as sodium bicarbonate in an effort to counteract the extreme acidosis that can occur when the weight is lifted off the patient.

Question 6: How does natural or normal cell death occur and what is it called?

Answer: Apoptosis is normal, genetically programmed cell death. Caspases are proteins that are activated by genes and lead to cell death. Proteins together with DNA undergo controlled degradation that allows them to be recycled by neighboring cells.

Question 7: What is the major difference between normal cell death and cell death due to hypoxia or other injury?

Answer: The major difference is that damaged cells from hypoxia or cellular toxins become necrotic and initiate an inflammatory response. Natural cell death is controlled and the body is able to eliminate cells in well-defined clusters rather than in a random fashion.

CASE STUDY ANSWERS

www.Paramedic.EMSzone.com

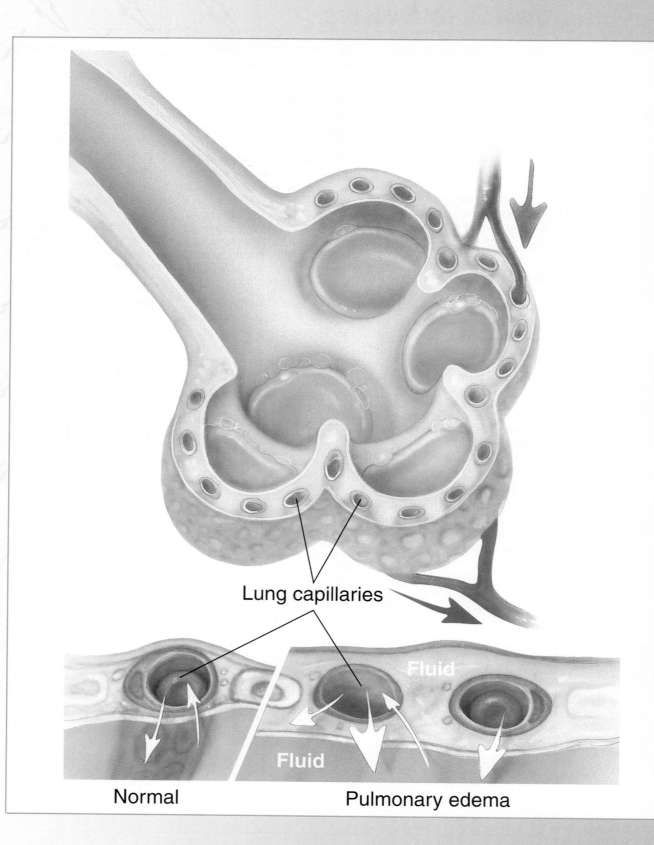

Lung capillaries

Normal

Fluid

Fluid

Pulmonary edema

The Cellular Environment

4

Objectives

Cognitive

1-6.4 Describe the cellular environment. (p 44)

Additional Objectives*

1. Describe the normal distribution of body fluids. (p 44)

2. Explain the basic mechanisms by which water and dissolved particles move across cell membranes. (p 46)

3. Define and explain osmosis. (p 46)

4. Explain the pathophysiology of edema and ascites. (p 48)

5. Define tonicity. (p 52)

6. Explain the role of the renin-angiotensin-aldosterone mechanism. (p 51)

7. List the causes and manifestations of hyponatremia, hypernatremia, hypokalemia, hyperkalemia, hypocalcemia, hypercalcemia, hypophosphatemia, hyperphosphatemia, hypomagnesemia, hypermagnesemia. (p 52–57, 60)

8. List five examples of extreme physical endurance activities. (p 58)

9. Describe the physiology of fluid balance during extreme physical endurance activities. (p 58)

10. List examples of athletes at risk for hyponatremia. (p 58)

11. Describe the pathophysiology and management of dehydration. (p 59–60)

12. Describe the pathophysiology and management of hyponatremia. (p 60)

13. Discuss the pathophysiology of postural hypotension. (p 61)

14. Define pH. (p 61)

15. Discuss normal acid-base balance and buffers. (p 61–62)

16. Define and explain differences between respiratory acidosis, respiratory alkalosis, metabolic acidosis, and metabolic alkalosis. (p 63–64)

*These are noncurriculum objectives.

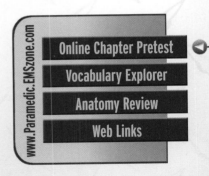

www.Paramedic.EMSzone.com

TECHNOLOGY

- Online Chapter Pretest
- Vocabulary Explorer
- Anatomy Review
- Web Links

Chapter FEATURES

- Case Studies
- Physiology Tips
- Medication Tips
- Paramedic Safety Tips
- Special Needs Tips
- Vital Vocabulary
- Prep Kit

Distribution of Body Fluids

The <u>cellular environment</u> refers to the distribution of cells, molecules, and fluids throughout the body. This environment changes with aging, disease, and injury (▼ **Figure 4-1**). Body fluids contain water, sodium, chloride, potassium, calcium, phosphorus, and magnesium. These chemicals move in and out of cells based on various factors to be discussed in this chapter. Another component of the cellular environment is acid-base balance.

The body consists primarily of water. About 50% to 70% of the total body weight is fluid and is referred to as the <u>total body water</u>. The average male is 60% fluid and the average female is 50% fluid. Body fluid is divided into two main compartments: <u>intracellular fluid</u> and <u>extracellular fluid</u>. Approximately 75% of the body's fluid is in the cells and is called intracellular fluid. The remaining 25% lies outside the cells and is called extracellular fluid. Extracellular fluid is further broken down into the fluid that is in-between the cells, called <u>interstitial fluid</u>, fluid inside the blood vessels, called <u>intravascular fluid</u>, lymph, and transcellular fluid. The interstitial fluid comprises approximately 10.5% of total body weight. An example of the relationship between the fluid in the cells and the diffusion of oxygen across the alveolar membrane through the interstitial fluid is illustrated in ▼ **Figure 4-2**. Circulation of the extracellular fluid is illustrated in ▶ **Figure 4-3**. <u>Transcellular fluid</u> includes cerebrospinal fluid, aqueous and vitreous humors in the eyes, synovial fluid in joints, serous fluid in body cavities (eg, pleural fluid), and glandular secretions.

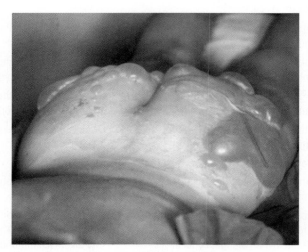

Figure 4-1 Extensive burns with marked leakage (extravasation) of fluid into the burned area leading to formation of large blisters.

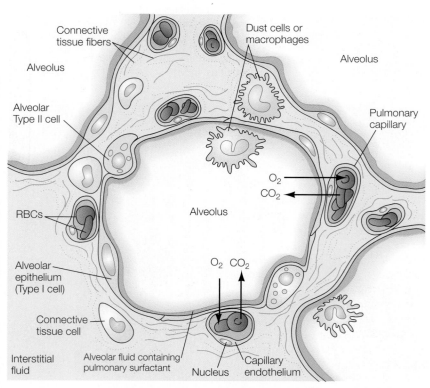

Figure 4-2 Close-up of the alveolus. Oxygen diffuses out of the alveolus into the capillary. Carbon dioxide diffuses in the opposite direction, entering the alveolar air that is expelled during exhalation. Note the location of the interstitial fluid within the figure.

Fluid and Water Balance

The average adult takes in about 2,500 mL of water a day. Sixty percent of this fluid intake occurs by drinking and another 30% comes from the water in foods, such as fruits. The remaining 10% is a byproduct of cellular metabolism.

Most water (60%) is lost in the form of urine; 28% is lost through the skin and lungs; 6% is lost in the feces; and 6% is lost through sweat. The amount of water lost through sweating is highly variable—in hot environmental conditions or during periods of rigorous exercise, it is possible to lose large amounts of fluid. During cooler temperatures or periods of relative inactivity, very little body water is lost by sweating.

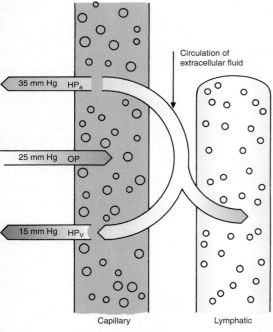

Figure 4-3 Factors regulating flow of fluid through the interstitial tissues. HP$_a$, hydrostatic pressure at the arterial end of the capillary. HP$_v$, hydrostatic pressure at the venous end of the capillary. OP, osmotic pressure. Hydrostatic pressure is the blood pressure in the vessel walls created by the heart beating, which pushes water out of the capillary into the interstitial space. Osmotic pressure is the measure of the tendency of water to move by osmosis across a membrane. Pressures are measured in millimeters of mercury (mm Hg). Fluid is forced from the arterial end of the capillary because the hydrostatic pressure exceeds the osmotic pressure. At the venous end of the capillary, the hydrostatic pressure is lower than the osmotic pressure and fluid returns. Lymphatic channels also collect some of the fluid forced from the capillaries by the hydrostatic pressure.

Case Study

Case Study, Part 1

Your unit is dispatched to a residence for a person who is sick. After establishing that the scene is safe, you find a 68-year-old woman lying on the couch. She appears to be alert, pale, and very weak. There is a bowl next to her that she has used to vomit in. Her husband tells you that she has been dizzy, nauseated, and vomiting for about an hour.

You introduce yourself to the patient and she answers you clearly. The patient's airway is clear and her breathing is nonlabored. She has an irregular distal pulse of 58 beats/min. She denies experiencing shortness of breath or any chest pain but has stomach cramps. You obtain her blood pressure and, as you expected, it is low.

Your general impression is that your patient is hypotensive and ALS will be needed. You ask a few more questions and discover that the events leading up to this episode included the patient mowing the lawn for 90 minutes in 92°F heat and high humidity.

Initial Assessment

Recording time
3 minutes

Appearance
Pale and weak

Level of consciousness
Alert

Airway
Open

Vital Signs

Pulse rate/quality
58 beats/min, irregular, weak

Blood pressure
90/40 mm Hg

Respiratory rate/depth
22 breaths/min, nonlabored

Question 1: What are the typical ways the body loses water, and how much water can be lost through sweating?

Question 2: What causes a hypotonic fluid deficit, and what are the signs and symptoms associated with it?

Question 3: How does the body monitor water balance?

CASE STUDY

Physiology Tip

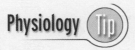

Sodium (Na$^+$), the major extracellular cation, is often lost along with water. This loss may affect nerve and muscle function as well as extracellular fluid volume.

Water and dissolved particles (<u>solutes</u>), such as molecules, move between cells as well as between blood vessels and connective tissues. The two general methods of movement are passive transport and active transport (▼ Figure 4-4). <u>Passive transport</u> includes:

- Diffusion – the movement of a substance from an area of higher concentration to an area of lower concentration.
- Facilitated diffusion – a transport molecule ("helper molecule") within the membrane helps the movement of a substance from areas of higher concentration to areas of lower concentration.
- Osmosis – the movement of a solvent, such as water, from an area of low solute concentration to one of high concentration through a selectively permeable membrane to equalize concentrations of a solute on both sides of the membrane.
- Filtration – the movement of water and a dissolved substance from an area of high pressure to an area of low pressure.

<u>Active transport</u> involves movement via "pumps" or transport molecules that require energy and move substances from an area of low concentration to an area of high concentration.

Water moves between intracellular and extracellular fluid by <u>osmosis</u>. Osmosis is the movement of water down its concentration gradient across a membrane. <u>Osmotic pressure</u> is the pressure that develops when two solutions of different concentrations are separated by a semipermeable membrane. Water moves from regions of low osmotic pressure to those of higher osmotic pressure (▶ Figure 4-5). When you compare two solutions, a solution with a higher solute concentration has a higher osmotic pressure and is referred to as a <u>hypertonic solution</u>. The solution with a lower solute concentration has a lower osmotic pressure and is referred to as a <u>hypotonic solution</u>. Solutions with equal solute concentrations are called <u>isotonic solutions</u> (ie, 0.9% NaCl or Lactated Ringer's solution).

The intracellular fluid volume is controlled by the large amount of proteins and organic compounds that cannot escape through the cell membrane and by the sodium-potassium (Na^+/K^+) membrane pump. Most of the intracellular substances are negatively charged and attract many positively charged ions, including potassium. Because all of these substances are osmotically active, they can pull water into the

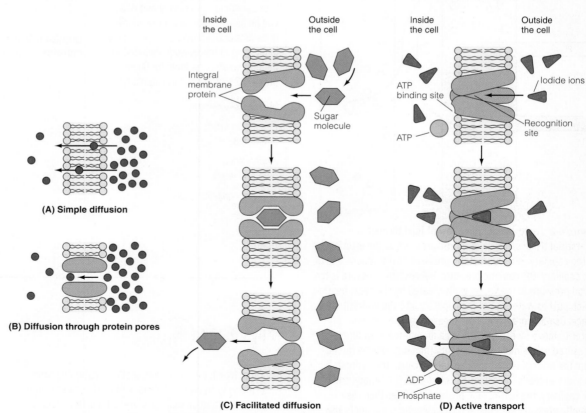

Figure 4-4 Methods of material transport through the cell wall. **A.** Simple diffusion. **B.** Diffusion through protein pores. **C.** Facilitated diffusion. **D.** Active transport.

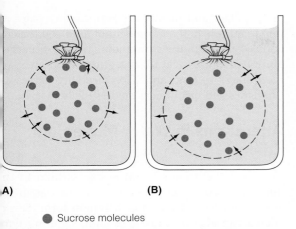

● Sucrose molecules

Figure 4-5 Osmosis is the diffusion of water molecules from a region of higher water concentration (or low solute concentration) to one of lower water concentration (or high solute concentration) across a selectively permeable membrane. **A.** To demonstrate the process, immerse a bag of sugar water in a solution of pure water. **B.** Water diffuses into the bag (toward the lower concentration), causing it to swell.

Physiology Tip

Some drugs, such as digitalis preparations, affect the sodium-potassium exchange pump. If toxic levels are reached in the blood, electrolyte imbalance leads to cardiac dysfunction and dysrhythmias.

cell until it ruptures. The pump is responsible for keeping this situation in check by continuously removing three Na^+ ions from the cell for every two K^+ ions that are moved back into the cell. If the pump is impaired due to insufficient potassium in the body, sodium accumulates and causes the cells to swell. The Na^+/K^+ pump must be functional as it is essential in the cell's electrical potential (▼ **Figure 4-6**).

Plasma makes up about 55% of the blood and is composed of 91% water and 9% plasma proteins.

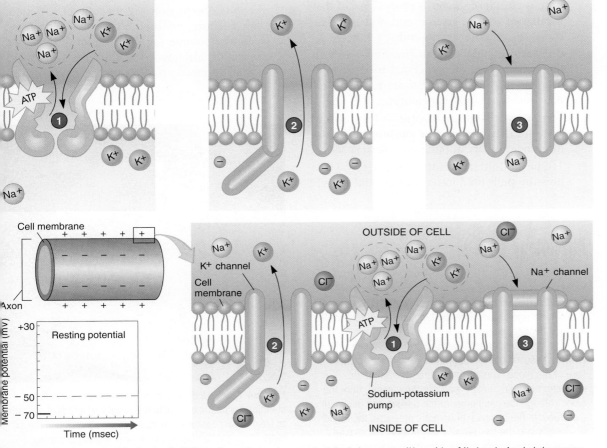

Figure 4-6 The cell's electrical potential. The cell membrane has an electrical charge on either side of it. A polarized state occurs when the inside of the nerve cell along its membrane is more negatively charged than the outside of the cell along the membrane. The difference in charge is the resting potential and is the basis for the transmission of signals by the nerves. ① indicates the sodium-potassium pump. ② indicates an open potassium channel. ③ indicates a closed sodium channel.

The plasma proteins include albumin (maintains osmotic pressure), globulin, fibrinogen, and prothrombin (assists with clotting).

Water moves between plasma and interstitial fluid based on conditions known as <u>Starling's law</u>, which is named after the English physiologist who originally described them, Dr. E. H. Starling. Under normal conditions, the amount of fluid filtering outward through the arterial ends of the capillaries equals the amount of fluid that is returned to the circulation by reabsorption at the venous ends of the capillaries. This equilibrium between the capillary and interstitial space is controlled by four forces: capillary hydrostatic pressure, capillary colloidal osmotic pressure, tissue hydrostatic pressure, and tissue colloidal osmotic pressure. The role of these four forces is as follows:

1. Capillary hydrostatic pressure – This is the pressure pushing water out of the capillary into the interstitial space. Because the pressure is higher on the arterial end than the venous end, more water is pushed out of the capillaries on the arterial end and more is reabsorbed on the venous end.
2. Capillary colloidal osmotic pressure – This is the osmotic pressure generated by dissolved proteins in the plasma that are too large to penetrate the capillary membrane.
3. Tissue hydrostatic pressure – This is the pressure that opposes the pushing of fluids from the capillary into the interstitial space.
4. Tissue colloidal osmotic pressure – This pressure pulls fluid into the interstitial space.

Physiology Tip

Several types of inhalation injuries (eg, smoke, chlorine) increase permeability in the lung capillaries. The result is rapid leakage of fluid into the lung spaces, a form of acute pulmonary edema.

The healthy liver produces the protein albumin, which is responsible for maintaining the osmotic pressure of the blood. This pressure directly affects the movement of fluid, mostly water in the plasma, from the blood through the capillaries to the tissues and back into the blood. In the absence of osmotic pressure, the blood fluid leaks into the tissues and stays there. Decreased plasma albumin levels reduce osmotic pressure, causing edema in the feet and ankles.

Capillary and membrane permeability plays an important role in the movement of fluid and the creation of edema in the surrounding tissues. If permeability increases, capillaries and membranes are more likely to leak, and if permeability decreases, capillaries and membranes are less likely to leak.

Alterations in Water Movement: Edema

<u>Edema</u> is the accumulation of excess fluid in the interstitial space. Peripheral edema, such as in the ankles and feet, is the most common form. Severe edema can also be caused by long-standing lymphatic obstruction (▼ **Figure 4-7**). If the patient is bedridden, edema may occur in the sacral area (sacral edema). <u>Ascites</u> is an abnormal accumulation of fluid in the peritoneal cavity.

The causes of edema include:

- Increased capillary pressure – arteriolar dilation (eg, allergic reactions, inflammation), venous obstruction (eg, hepatic obstruction, heart failure, or thrombophlebitis), increased vascular volume (eg, heart failure), increased levels of adrenocortical hormones, premenstrual sodium retention, pregnancy, environ-

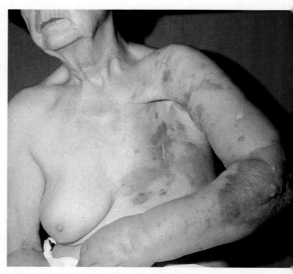

Figure 4-7 Severe edema of the arm resulting from long-standing lymphatic obstruction. Patient had a radical operation to treat breast cancer many years earlier. Scarring in the axilla blocked lymphatic drainage from arm, leading to chronic edema. The dark discolored areas in the skin of the chest wall and upper limb are caused by a malignant tumor of the lymphatic vessels (lymphangiosarcoma), which sometimes complicates chronic lymphedema.

Physiology Tip

The clinical manifestations of edema may be local at an injury site or generalized. Patients may have pulmonary edema for cardiac reasons, or edema may present following near drowning or a narcotic overdose. Excess fluid in the lungs (eg, acute pulmonary edema) impairs the diffusion of oxygen into pulmonary capillaries, making the patient hypoxic (▼ **Figure 4-8**). Patients can literally drown in their own fluids if proper medications are not administered.

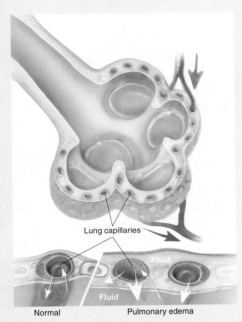

Figure 4-8 Pulmonary edema develops as the result of fluid build-up within the lungs. The edema causes swelling and leads to impaired ventilation.

Case Study

Case Study, Part 2

You give the patient oxygen by nasal cannula; this way, if she vomits, a mask will not be in the way. As you attach her to your monitor and begin a focused physical examination, you discover that the patient has a history of hypertension and takes a beta-blocker. The beta-blocker could explain why her heart rate is slow despite having other signs of shock. Also, this past week she started taking a water pill for swelling in her legs, which may be contributing to the complaints today. She has no allergies to medications and has never had a stroke, heart attack, or surgeries.

The focused physical exam reveals clear lung sounds; pale, warm, moist skin; a soft, nontender abdomen, despite the cramping; mild pitting edema in her lower legs; and dizziness that worsens when she tries to sit up. Before you move the patient to the ambulance, you begin an IV of normal saline.

Focused Physical Assessment

Recording time
5 minutes

Lung sounds
Clear bilaterally

Signs
Skin is pale, warm, and moist.
Pedal edema present in the lower legs

Neurologic exam
Speech is clear; equal strength in all extremities

Diagnostic Tools

Electrocardiogram
Sinus bradycardia with premature ventricular contractions

SpO$_2$
99%

Question 4: How can diuretic therapy (water pills) affect the body's electrolyte balance?

Question 5: What type of solution is normal saline classified as: isotonic, hypotonic, or hypertonic? Why is this solution a first choice for use in the management of dehydration?

CASE STUDY

mental heat stress, and the effects of gravity from prolonged standing.

- Decreased colloidal osmotic pressure in the capillaries – decreased production of plasma proteins (eg, liver disease, starvation, or severe protein deficiency), increased loss of plasma proteins (eg, protein-losing kidney diseases, extensive burns).

- Lymphatic vessel obstruction due to infection, disease of the lymphatic structures or their removal (eg, mastectomy and removal of lymph nodes may lead to edema in the upper extremity).

Fluid and Electrolyte Balance

Water balance in the body is maintained through a combination of many different factors. Normally, the thirst mechanism and release of <u>antidiuretic hormone (ADH)</u> are the most important (▶ **Figure 4-9**). The renin-angiotensin-aldosterone system also plays a role in water homeostasis. The body's state of hydration is monitored continuously by three different types of receptors located in the brain, blood vessels, and kidneys:

1. <u>Osmoreceptors</u> are sensory receptors that monitor extracellular fluid osmolarity. Sensors

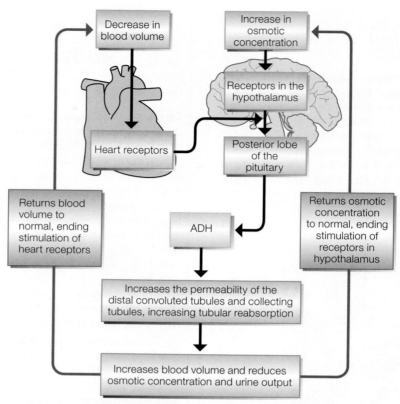

Figure 4-9 Antidiuretic hormone (ADH) secretion is under the control of the hypothalamus. When the osmotic concentration of the blood rises, receptors in the hypothalamus detect the change and trigger the release of ADH from the posterior lobe of the pituitary. Detectors in the heart also respond to changes in the blood volume. When it drops, they send signals to the brain, causing the release of ADH.

Physiology Tip

When edematous tissue is compressed with a finger, the fluid is pushed aside, causing an impression or "pit" that gradually refills. Referred to as pitting edema, this condition can be significant in patients who have chronic heart failure.

for these receptors are located primarily in the hypothalamus. When the extracellular fluid osmolarity is too high, they stimulate the production of ADH (see below).

2. **Volume-sensitive receptors** are receptors located in the atria that respond to stretch. When the intravascular fluid volume increases, the atria are stretched, leading to the release of natriuretic proteins (see below).

3. **Baroreceptors** are receptors found primarily in the carotid artery, aorta, and kidneys, which are sensitive to changes in the blood pressure.

The most potent stimulation for the release of ADH is an increase in blood osmolarity. Changes in blood volume and blood pressure are less of a stimulus. When osmolarity increases, the pituitary gland releases ADH, also known as *vasopressin*. ADH stimulates the kidneys to resorb water, decreasing the osmolarity of the blood.

Sodium and Chloride Balance

Sodium is the most common cation, or positively charged ion, in the body. The average adult has 60 mEq of sodium for each kilogram of body weight (2.2 lb = 1 kg). Most of the body's sodium is found in the extracellular fluid, but a small amount is found in the intracellular fluid. Intracellular sodium is transported out of the cell by the sodium-potassium pump because a resting cell membrane is relatively impermeable to sodium. Sodium also plays an important role in the regulation of the body's acid-base balance (sodium bicarbonate buffer system).

Sodium is taken in with foods. As little as 500 mg per day meets the body's needs. In the United States, studies have shown that the average adult

Physiology Tip

Normally, only about 10% of the sodium is lost through the skin and gastrointestinal tract. However, the loss of sodium due to diarrhea, vomiting, extensive burns, or fistula drainage can be considerable. Sweat loss increases greatly with vigorous exercise and exposure to a hot environment. A person sweating profusely can lose 30 g of sodium per day. This is why some exercise physiologists recommend that athletes consume sports drinks that replace electrolytes, such as sodium, when engaged in lengthy training.

ingests between 6 and 15 g of sodium per day. Sodium regulation occurs in the kidneys. When there is an excess of sodium, it is excreted into the urine. When the body sodium levels are low, the kidneys resorb sodium.

Sodium is regulated primarily by the **renin-angiotensin-aldosterone system (RAAS)** and by natriuretic proteins. The RAAS is a complex feedback mechanism responsible for the kidney's regulation of sodium in the body. Renin is a protein that is released by the kidney into the bloodstream in response to changes in blood pressure, blood flow, the amount of sodium in the tubular fluid, and the glomerular filtration rate. A **natriuretic protein** is a protein that increases the rate of excretion of sodium in the urine.

When renin is released it converts the plasma protein angiotensinogen to angiotensin I. In the lung, angiotensin I is converted rapidly to **angiotensin II** by an angiotensin-converting enzyme. Angiotensin II is responsible for stimulating sodium resorption by the renal tubules. It also constricts the renal blood vessels, slowing kidney blood flow and decreasing the glomerular filtration rate. As a result, less sodium is filtered into the urine and more is resorbed in the blood. The relationship of the kidneys in the regulation of the blood pressure and blood volume is illustrated in ▶ **Figure 4-10**.

Angiotensin II is also responsible for stimulating the secretion of the adrenal hormone **aldosterone**. Aldosterone acts on the kidneys to increase the reabsorption of sodium into the blood and the elimination of potassium in the urine. In addition to angiotensin II, three other factors stimulate aldosterone release:

1. Increased extracellular potassium levels
2. Decreased extracellular sodium levels

Case Study

Case Study, Part 3

You keep the patient lying down and elevate her legs. After the patient has been moved to the ambulance and transport has begun, you perform an ongoing assessment. The patient's symptoms have not changed in the past few minutes. It is important to observe for changes in mental status and airway patency.

While you obtain another set of vital signs and repeat the neurologic exam, the patient tells you that she mows her lawn every week and this type of thing has never happened before. With positioning and IV fluid administration her blood pressure has risen. The pulse is less irregular now and respirations remain adequate.

Ongoing Assessment

Recording time
15 minutes

Appearance
Weak

Level of consciousness
Alert

Airway
Open

Lung sounds
Clear

Vital Signs

Pulse rate/quality
60 beats/min and slightly irregular

Blood pressure
106/54 mm Hg

Respiratory rate/depth
18 breaths/min, nonlabored

Diagnostic Tools

Electrocardiogram
Normal sinus rhythm at a rate of 60 beats/min, with occasional premature ventricular contractions

Question 6: How does water move between intracellular fluid and extracellular fluid?

Question 7: What protein and what type of pressure are responsible for causing edema in the lower extremities of this patient?

3. Release of adrenocorticotropic hormone (ACTH) from the pituitary gland (▶ **Figure 4-11**).

Activation of the RAAS leads to retention of sodium and water. To maintain balance when there is too much sodium and water, the body produces natriuretic proteins, which inhibit ADH and promote excretion of sodium and water by the kidneys.

The interaction of ADH, renin, angiotensin II, aldosterone (as illustrated in ▶ **Figure 4-12**), and the natriuretic proteins regulate sodium and fluid levels in the body.

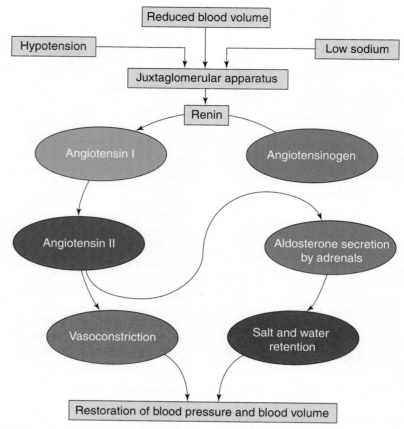

Figure 4-10 Role of the kidneys in regulation of blood pressure and blood volume.

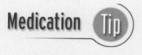

Medication Tip

IV fluids may be isotonic (0.9% NaCl), hypertonic (mannitol), or hypotonic (D$_5$W) to the blood.

Chloride is an important anion, or negatively charged ion, that, when combined with sodium, makes ordinary table salt. When placed in water, the compound will separate into its original ionic form (▶ **Figure 4-13**). It assists in regulating the acid-base balance, especially the pH of the stomach, and is involved in the osmotic pressure of the extracellular fluid. Table salt, milk, eggs, and meats all contain chloride. It is often the case that, where sodium goes, chloride follows.

Alterations in Sodium, Chloride, and Water Balance

Changes in water content can cause a cell to shrink or swell. Tonicity refers to the tension exerted on a cell due to water movement across the cell membrane. Solutions that body cells are exposed to are classified as isotonic, hypotonic, or hypertonic. Cells that are placed in an isotonic solution, which has the same osmolarity as intracellular fluid (280 mOsm/L), neither shrink nor swell. When cells are placed in a hypertonic solution, which has a greater osmolarity than intracellular fluid, water is pulled out of the cells and they shrink. When cells are placed in a hypotonic solution, which has a lower osmolarity than intracellular fluid, they swell.

An isotonic fluid deficit is a decrease in extracellular fluid with proportionate losses of sodium and water. An isotonic fluid excess represents a proportionate increase in both sodium and water in the extracellular fluid compartment. Common causes include kidney, heart, or liver failure. A hypertonic fluid deficit is caused by excess body water loss without a proportionate sodium loss (a relative water loss exists). The result, clinically, is hypernatremia, defined as a serum sodium level that is above 148 mEq/L and a serum osmolarity greater than 295 mOsm/kg.

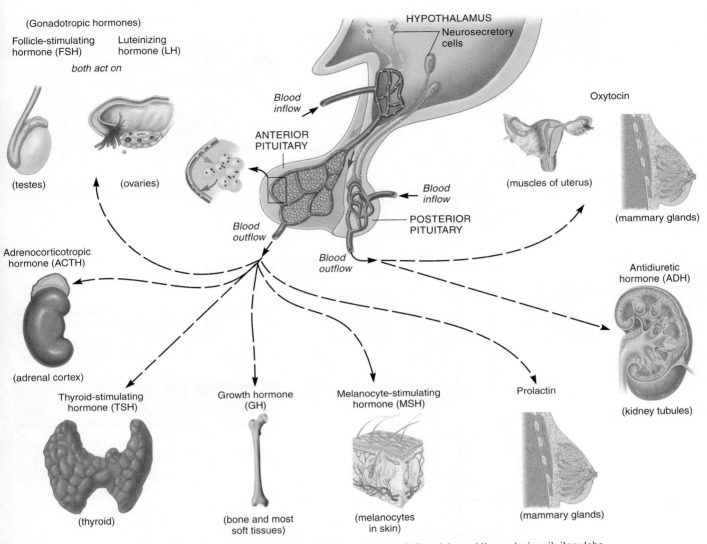

Figure 4-11 The pituitary gland secretes hormones from its two portions, the anterior pituitary lobe and the posterior pituitary lobe.

Manifestations depend on the serum sodium level. When dehydration exists, orthostatic hypotension and decreased urine output (oliguria) are common. Hyperthermia, delirium, and coma may be seen with very high levels (eg, >160 mEq/L).

A hypotonic fluid deficit is caused by excessive sodium loss with less water loss (a relative water excess exists). The result is <u>hyponatremia</u>, a serum sodium level that is below 135 mEq/L and a serum osmolarity that is less than 280 mOsm/kg. Causes of either hypernatremia or hyponatremia may include excess sweating from hot environmental conditions or exercise, or gastrointestinal losses through vomiting, diarrhea, inappropriate intravenous fluids, or diuretics. Some of these patients have nausea and headaches, while others can go on to develop seizures and coma. Clinical findings typically depend not only on the absolute sodium level, but

Medication Tip

A hypertonic solution, such as mannitol, contains more solute than the interstitial or tissue fluid in the brain. This causes excess fluid to be drawn into the blood, decreasing swelling within the brain.

also the time period over which the abnormality developed. Patients who become hyponatremic over a period of days tend to have fewer symptoms than those whose conditions develop the abnormality acutely. Hyponatremia is discussed in further detail later in this chapter.

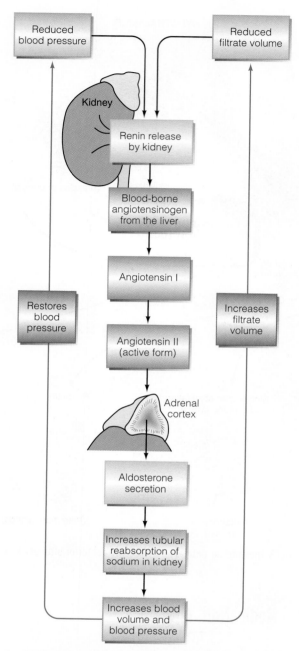

Figure 4-12 Aldosterone secretion. Aldosterone is released by the adrenal cortex. Its release, however, is stimulated by a chain of events that begins in the kidney.

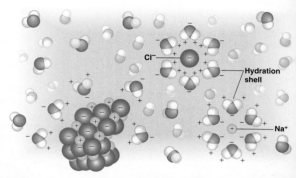

Figure 4-13 Sodium placed into water will separate into its original ionic form.

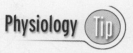

Physiology Tip

Normal lab values vary from laboratory to laboratory. All lab values used in this text are approximations. The normal range for lab test results is usually printed on the report form and is listed in ▼ Table 4-1.

Table 4-1 *Normal Reference Serum Laboratory Values of Electrolytes*	
Calcium	8.5–10.5 mg/100 mL
Chloride	100–106 mEq/L
Iron	50–150 µg/100 mL (higher in males)
Magnesium	1.5–2.0 mEq/L
Potassium	3.5–5.0 mEq/L
Sodium	135–145 mEq/L

Alterations in Potassium, Calcium, Phosphate, and Magnesium Balance

Potassium is the major intracellular cation and is critical to many functions of the cell. Potassium is necessary for neuromuscular control, regulation of the three types of muscles (skeletal, smooth, and cardiac), acid-base balance, intracellular enzyme reactions, and maintenance of intracellular osmolar-ity. Potassium (K+) levels may be normal, low (hypokalemia), or elevated (hyperkalemia).

Hypokalemia is defined as a decreased serum potassium level. Common causes include decreased potassium intake, potassium shifts into the cells (eg, insulin, alkalosis, beta-adrenergic stimulation such as with epinephrine), renal potassium losses (eg, increased aldosterone activity, diuretics), and extra-renal potassium losses (eg, vomiting, diarrhea, laxatives).

Muscular weakness, fatigue, and muscle cramps are the most frequent complaints in mild to moderate hypokalemia. Flaccid paralysis, hyporeflexia, and tetany may occur with very low levels of potassium (<2.5 mEq/L). The ECG shows decreased amplitude and broadening of T waves, prominent U waves, premature ventricular contractions (and other dysrhythmias, such as torsades de pointes), and depressed ST segments.

Physiology Tip

Treatment of hyperkalemia depends on the clinical presentation. Calcium administered intravenously immediately antagonizes cardiac conduction abnormalities. Bicarbonate, insulin, and albuterol shift potassium into the cells during a 15- to 30-minute period.

Physiology Tip

In the presence of tetany, arrhythmias, or seizures, 10% IV calcium gluconate (10 to 20 mL) administered over 10 to 15 minutes is indicated. Oral calcium and vitamin D preparations are used in more moderate or asymptomatic cases. Uses of IV calcium in the field: suspected hypocalcemia, hyperkalemia with ECG changes or dysrhythmias, treatment of known calcium-blocker overdose.

Hyperkalemia is defined as an elevated serum potassium level. Common causes include spurious (repeated fist clenching during phlebotomy, with release of potassium from forearm muscles; specimen drawn from an arm with a potassium infusion); decreased excretion (renal failure, drugs that inhibit potassium excretion [spironolactone, angiotensin-converting enzyme inhibitors, nonsteroidal anti-inflammatory drugs (NSAIDs)]); shifts of potassium from within the cell (eg, burns, metabolic acidosis, insulin deficiency); and excessive intake of potassium.

An elevated serum potassium concentration interferes with normal neuromuscular function, leading to muscle weakness and, rarely, flaccid paralysis. ECG changes occur in less than half of patients with a serum potassium level greater than 6.5 mEq/L and include peaked T waves, widening of the QRS complex, and dysrhythmias (eg, ventricular tachycardia).

Although acute hypokalemia can be treated with IV potassium supplementation, this treatment is rarely undertaken in the out-of-hospital setting.

The majority of the body's calcium is found in the bone. Calcium provides strength and stability for the collagen and ground substance that forms the matrix of the skeletal system. Calcium enters the body through the gastrointestinal tract and is absorbed from the intestine in a process that is dependent on vitamin D. Vitamin D is mostly attained from exposure to sunlight. It is then stored in the bone and ultimately excreted by the kidney. Calcium levels may be normal, low (hypocalcemia), or elevated (hypercalcemia), and their effects are illustrated in ▶ Figure 4-14.

Hypocalcemia is defined as a decreased serum calcium level. Causes of hypocalcemia include decreased intake or absorption (eg, malabsorption, vitamin D deficit); increased loss (eg, alcoholism, diuretic therapy); and endocrine disease (eg, hypoparathyroidism, sepsis).

Common symptoms reflect increased excitation of the neuromuscular and cardiovascular systems.

Spasm of skeletal muscle causes cramps and tetany. Laryngospasm with stridor can obstruct the airway. Convulsions can occur as well as abnormal sensations (paresthesias) of the lips and extremities. Prolongation of the QT interval predisposes to the development of ventricular arrhythmias.

Hypercalcemia is defined as an increased serum calcium level. Common causes include increased intake or absorption (eg, excess antacid ingestion); endocrine disorders (eg, primary hyperparathyroidism, adrenal insufficiency); neoplasms (eg, cancers); and miscellaneous (eg, diuretics, sarcoidosis).

Common symptoms are constipation and frequent urination (polyuria). Stupor, coma, and renal failure may develop in severe hypercalcemia.

Phosphate is primarily an intracellular anion and is essential to many body functions. Phosphate levels may be normal, low (hypophosphatemia), or elevated (hyperphosphatemia).

Treatment of the underlying cause, when known, is the mainstay of dealing with hypercalcemia. Acutely, volume repletion with boluses of 0.45% or 0.9% normal saline may be helpful.

Hypophosphatemia is characterized by a decrease in serum phosphate levels. Causes include:

- Decreased supply or absorption (eg, starvation, malabsorption, blocked absorption [alumin-containing antacids])
- Excessive loss (eg, diuretics, hyperparathyroidism, hyperthyroidism, alcoholism)
- Intracellular shift of phosphorus (eg, administration of glucose, anabolic steroids, oral contraceptives, respiratory alkalosis, salicylate poisoning)
- Electrolyte abnormalities (eg, hypercalcemia, hypomagnesemia, metabolic acidosis)
- Abnormal losses followed by inadequate repletion (eg, diabetic ketoacidosis, chronic alcoholism)

LOW BLOOD CALCIUM			HIGH BLOOD CALCIUM	
Increase PTH secretion and calcitriol formation	Thyroid/Parathyroid		**Secrete calcitonin**	**Decrease PTH secretion and calcitriol formation**
Parathyroid gland secretes PTH. Increased PTH levels stimulate calcitriol (vitamin D$_3$) production in the kidney	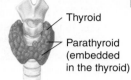 Thyroid — Parathyroid (embedded in the thyroid)		Thyroid gland secretes calcitonin	PTH formation slows and PTH levels drop. Decreased PTH levels slow calcitriol formation
Absorb more dietary calcium	Small intestine		**Absorb less dietary calcium**	
Calcitriol increases intestinal absorption of calcium and phosphorus			No major effect – calcitonin slightly inhibits calcium absorption	Decreased calcitriol slows intestinal absorption of calcium and phosphorus
Retain calcium	Kidney		**Excrete calcium**	
PTH and calcitriol increase calcium reabsorption in the kidney, thus decreasing calcium excretion			No major effect – calcitonin slightly increases calcium excretion	Decreased PTH and calcitriol levels increase calcium excretion
Move calcium from bone to bloodstream	Bone		**Move calcium from bloodstream to bone**	
PTH and calcitriol work together to stimulate osteoclast activity. The osteoclasts resorb bone, releasing calcium into the bloodstream			Calcitonin inhibits the activity of osteoclasts, shifting the balance toward the deposition of calcium in bone	Decreased PTH and calcitriol levels slow osteoclast activity and breakdown of bone
RAISE BLOOD CALCIUM			**LOWER BLOOD CALCIUM**	

Figure 4-14 Regulating blood calcium levels. Calcitonin has only a weak effect on calcium ion concentration. It is fast acting, but any decrease in calcium ion concentration triggers the release of parathyroid hormone (PTH), which almost completely overrides the calcitonin effect. In prolonged calcium excess or deficiency, the parathyroid mechanism is the most powerful hormonal mechanism for maintaining normal blood calcium levels.

Symptoms include muscle weakness, decreased deep tendon reflexes, mental obtundation, and confusion. Weakness is common. Acute, severe hypophosphatemia can lead to acute hemolytic anemia and susceptibility to infection. Muscle death (rhabdomyolysis) may also occur. Treatment involves oral replenishment.

Hyperphosphatemia is defined as an increased serum phosphate level. Causes include:

- Massive load of phosphate into the extracellular fluid (eg, excess vitamin D, laxatives, or enemas containing phosphate, IV phosphate supplements, chemotherapy, metabolic acidosis)

- Decreased excretion into the urine (eg, renal failure, hypoparathyroidism, excessive growth hormone [acromegaly])

Symptoms vary widely from patient to patient and may include tremor, paresthesia, hyporeflexia, confusion, seizures, muscle weakness, stupor, and coma. Treatment of the underlying cause and of accompanying hypocalcemia is the most common therapeutic approach.

Magnesium is the second most abundant intracellular cation, after potassium. About 50% of the body's magnesium is stored in the bones, 49% is contained in the body cells, and the remaining 1% is in the extracellular fluid. Serum levels may be normal, low (hypomagnesemia), or high (hypermagnesemia).

<u>Hypomagnesemia</u> is defined as a decreased serum magnesium level. Causes include:

- Diminished absorption or intake (eg, malabsorption, chronic diarrhea, laxative abuse, malnutrition)
- Increased renal loss (eg, diuretics, hyperaldosteronism, hypercalcemia, volume expansion)
- Others (eg, diabetes, respiratory alkalosis, pregnancy)

Common symptoms are weakness, muscle cramps, and tremor. There is marked neuromuscular and central nervous system hyperirritability with tremors and jerking. There may be hypertension, tachycardia, and ventricular arrhythmias. In some patients, confusion and disorientation are prominent features. Treatment consists of IV fluids containing magnesium.

<u>Hypermagnesemia</u> is defined as an increased serum magnesium level. The cause is almost always the result of kidney insufficiency and the inability to excrete what has been taken in from food or drugs, especially antacids and laxatives. Symptoms include muscle weakness, decreased deep tendon reflexes, mental obtundation, and confusion. Weakness is common. There may be respiratory muscle paralysis or cardiac arrest.

Heat Stress from Extreme Physical Activity: Proper Hydration

This section is intended to discuss the physiology and pathophysiology of the conditions that may occur if a person is not properly hydrating. Paramedics are often asked to stand-by or respond to large-scale sporting events in their community. This material is designed to complement current paramedic training materials by discussing misconceptions about hydration as well as the current theories for assessment and management of the athlete. Paramedics may encounter patients who engage in activities that result in similar stresses to the body, such as heavy work for lengthy periods of time in very hot conditions or firefighting; for this reason, it can be instructive to learn how athletes are affected by extreme physical activity and how they prepare for the worst challenges.

In the past three decades there has been a tremendous increase in the number of athletes participating in endurance activities. Within the United

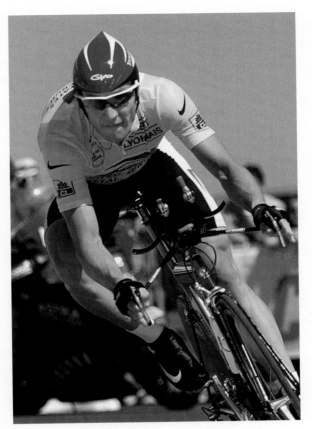

Figure 4-15 One of the best known modern endurance athletes is Lance Armstrong, seven-time winner of the Tour de France and a cancer survivor. Proper hydration, conditioning, and nutrition have been instrumental in his tremendous success as an athlete.

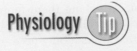

Physiology Tip

Calcium acts as an antagonist to magnesium and may be given intravenously as calcium chloride, 500 mg or more at a rate of 100 mg/min. Patients may require hemodialysis.

States alone, the USA Track and Field estimates there are now 30 million adult runners. The popularity of road biking has increased in the United States due in a large part to the enormous success of Lance Armstrong and his team in the past seven Tour de France races (▲ **Figure 4-15**). In 1982, Julie Moss crawled across the finish line of the Ironman Triathlon competition and inspired hundreds of athletes to take up the sport with her mantra: "Just finishing the Ironman is a victory!" The International

Olympic Committee agreed to debut the triathlon event to the 2000 Sidney Summer Olympics, and this has expanded the popularity of the sport into many communities across the United States.

Examples of extreme physical (endurance) activities include:

- Running marathons (26.2 miles) or ultra-marathons (more than 26.2 miles)
- Ironman (swim 2.4 miles, then bike 112 miles, then run 26.2 miles) or Half Ironman competitions (swim 1.2 miles, then bike 56 miles, then run 13.1 miles)
- Time trials (long sprints)
- Triathlon Olympic distance (swim 0.9 miles, then bike 24.8 miles, then run 6.2 miles)
- Criterium road races (approximately 25- to 75-mile road bike events) and Century Rides (100-mile bike ride)
- Stage races (multiple day races of varying lengths and difficulty levels, such as the Tour of Georgia) and 24-hour off-road races

Physiology

For a 150-lb male (approximately 70 kg), it is expected that his kidneys will produce 1 L of water (in the form of urine) per hour. Add to this approximately 1 L of fluid loss from sweating, and this person then loses approximately 2 L of fluid per hour.

However, while running or participating in vigorous exercise, research has shown that the "sweat rates" drop to about 300 mL per hour and urine production diminishes. This situation is actually more pronounced in women, making them more prone to fluid overload when drinking too much fluid. Studies have shown that women only need to drink approximately 2.5 kg of fluid to cause death.

In addition to concerns over sweat rates and urine production, in a recent study the researchers found that 80% of runners they surveyed took analgesics. More than 88% of the respondents reported using NSAIDs such as naprosyn (naproxen) and ibuprofen. These drugs are known to impair the body's ability to excrete water, which can, theoretically, contribute to the patient's hyponatremia risk. Acetaminophen has been shown to be safe.

The real issue here is a balance between fluid loss and fluid intake to help the body avoid the extreme conditions of dehydration or hyponatremia. Dehydration can result from excessive body fluid loss, and hyponatremia can result from an overall dangerously low level of the body's electrolyte sodium. Normal sodium levels should be between 138 and 142 mEq/L. This condition is exacerbated by the combination of salt loss from sweating and dilution of the remaining salt within the body by an intake of an excessive amount of fluid.

In addition, one theory suggests that the body's hormonal response to the muscle injury from endurance sports can play a significant role in hyponatremia. Analysis of the blood samples from runners who died of hyponatremia seem to show that elevated levels of interleukin-6 released during rhabdomyolysis (muscle tissue breakdown) stimulate the brain to release arginine vasopressin, an antidiuretic hormone, that in turn causes the kidneys to stop secreting water.

In the past, endurance sports enthusiasts have been told to "Drink up so you are ahead of the curve and never feel thirsty." The theory was that thirst is a sensation that is often felt only after a person is already dehydrated. The assumption, which has yet to be proven in the medical literature, was that dehydration and hyperthermia, two conditions that can be prevented by fluid ingestion, should be avoided at all costs. Some athletes have interpreted the fluid mantra to mean: "Drink to the point of hearing the fluid slosh in your stomach as you run."

Fluid intake is usually not a problem for elite athletes because they complete marathons in 126 to 140 minutes, giving them little time to actually drink too much. However, as running has increased in popularity, more and more marathon participants are crossing the finish line in over 5 hours, which gives them plenty of time to overhydrate. The fluid overload leads to hyponatremia, which can lead to life-threatening conditions such as brain swelling, seizures, respiratory arrest, and cardiac dysrhythmias.

Who Is at Risk for Hyponatremia?

- Men and women are affected equally; however, women are more likely to be severely affected.
- Slower runners, who take over 4 to 4.5 hours to complete their activity and continue to drink too much fluid during the event.
- People on low-sodium diets.
- People whose extreme exercise will take over 4 to 4.5 hours to complete and who do not replace sodium during the event (ie, by drinking a sports drink, eating pretzels).
- People who overhydrate before, during, and after exercise.
- People who are "salty sweaters," as indicated by white residue on their skin and clothing after exercise.

How Can Hyponatremia Be Prevented?

Proper hydration is the key to prevention of hyponatremia. If you are going to engage in an extreme activity, such as roofing a house on a hot, humid day or fighting a fire in heavy turnout clothing, it is helpful to understand how athletes learn to properly balance their hydration to avoid the extreme conditions (ie, dehydration or hyponatremia). The following suggestions should be helpful:

- When doing strenuous exercise for more than an hour, drink a sports drink that contains more than water (ie, carbohydrates and electrolytes such as sodium). Athletes who are training for a long race always check to see which specific drink will be available and train with that beverage. If the drink does not work well for you, consider carrying your own sports drink and alternate drinking your sports drink and their water. It is strongly suggested that any water offered by spectators be used for cooling your body and not for drinking in order to limit pathogen intake.

- A "drinking plan" for a lengthy event should focus on drinking as often as desired (when thirsty) provided intake does not exceed 800 mL/h for events less than 4 hours and no more than 600 mL/h for greater than 4 hours.

- To become "tuned in" to these volumes of fluid, athletes "measure" their fluid intake in various size cups during their training. This helps them estimate how much fluid the event cups hold.

- Athletes are told to not take any NSAIDs within 24 hours prior to the event and to wait for a minimum of 6 hours after completing the event to begin taking NSAIDs.

- Finally, if the athlete is a salty sweater, consider sodium supplements or eating salted pretzels during the event as long as the stomach can tolerate it.

- Athletes are instructed to determine their rate of sweat loss, in advance of the event, using the Self-Testing Program for Optimal Hydration developed by the USA Track and Field.

Pathophysiology of Dehydration and Hyponatremia

Dehydration

Dehydration is an acute and significant loss of fluid stores within the body that can lead to a state of hypohydration that alters the body's normal physiologic functions. This condition can increase the heart rate and cause sweating and the endurance capacity of the muscles to be detrimentally altered as the volume of fluid loss reaches critical levels. Dehydration can also lead to orthostatic hypotension as well as contribute to heat disorders by inhibiting the vasodilatation that is essential in thermolysis. During exercise, when sweat losses exceed the fluid intake, dehydration ensues. Mild dehydration, involving 1% to 2% of the total body weight is likely and not of concern. Fluid losses causing a body weight decrease in excess of 3% may require rehydration either orally or by IV. If a patient has a fluid loss that represents a total body weight loss of 7%, they may be considered to be in decompensated shock and should be managed promptly.

The clinical manifestations of dehydration include:

- Neurologic findings such as headache or mental status changes
- Weakness, dizziness, and severe fatigue
- Personality changes and irritability
- Gastrointestinal distress, such as vomiting, nausea, abdominal cramps, and decreased urine output, which often manifests as very dark-colored urine
- Muscle cramps
- Abnormal chills
- Heat flush
- Weak, rapid pulse
- Hypotension or normal blood pressure

The management concerns for dehydration include:

- Conduct an initial assessment (assess mental status, airway, breathing, and circulation, and determine priority). Manage the patient's ABCs as you locate any life-threats.
- Obtain a set of baseline vital signs right away (pulse, respiration, blood pressure, body temperature, and weight)!
- If the patient is dizzy or lightheaded, place the patient in the Trendelenberg position.
- Rule out ischemic chest pain and lethal dysrhythmias (with history and a 12-lead ECG for ST-segment elevation in two consecutive precordial leads; note that acute myocardial infarction may be difficult to rule out in the field). Rule out hypoglycemia in the patient with a history of diabetes (with a fingerstick

and glucometer). Rule out a stroke or transient ischemic attack (by assessing mental status and administering the Cincinnati Prehospital Stroke Scale). Rule out seizure activity, and rule out an elevated body temperature.

- Take another set of vital signs and consider these fluid guidelines:
  - Generally, the patient should drink a pint of electrolyte replacement fluid for every pound of documented weight lost, if he or she can tolerate it.
  - If the patient's hypotension, dizziness, and nausea continue after 10 minutes in the Trendelenberg position, consider starting a large-bore IV and administering a fluid challenge of 500 mL of normal saline. Obtain blood samples to determine the patient's serum sodium level.
  - Reassess the patient every 15 minutes and determine the need for transport to an emergency department or release of the patient once symptoms have subsided and vital signs are normal. This decision should be made with the consultation of medical control.

Hyponatremia

Although hyponatremia is rare, it can be very serious and sometimes deadly if not managed appropriately. The clinical manifestations of hyponatremia include:

- Neurologic findings, such as a throbbing headache, lack of coordination, seizure, and pathologic reflexes
- Weakness, dizziness, and severe fatigue
- Personality changes such as depression or apathy
- Mental status changes, such as confusion, apprehension and a feeling of impending doom, and lethargy, stupor, or coma
- Rales and crackles in all lung fields
- Gastrointestinal distress, such as anorexia, nausea, or vomiting, abdominal cramps, a bloated stomach, and diarrhea
- Pitting edema of hands and feet
- Rapid weight gain
- The blood pressure can be hypotensive, normotensive, or hypertensive.

Patients can present with serum sodium levels of mild (130 to 135 mmol/L) to moderate (124 to 129 mmol/L) to critical (<124 mmol/L). Typically, symptoms of *critical patients* include an altered mental status, vomiting, delirium, seizures, normotension to hypertension, normal body temperature, lung sounds of rales and crackles in all fields, and pathologic reflexes.

Assessment and Management of Hyponatremia

Until recently, athletes who arrived at the medical aide station with headache, nausea, or vomiting would routinely be given IV fluids. However, for the patient with hyponatremia, this treatment would not be the most appropriate because it might further dilute what little sodium the patient has left.

Assessment and management of the hyponatremic patient include the following:

- Conduct an initial assessment (assess mental status, airway, breathing, and circulation, and determine priority). Manage the patient's ABCs as you locate any life-threats.
- Obtain a set of baseline vital signs right away (pulse, respiration, blood pressure, body temperature, and weight)!
- If the patient is dizzy or lightheaded, place the patient in the Trendelenberg position.
- Rule out ischemic chest pain and lethal dysrhythmias (with history and a 12-lead ECG for ST-segment elevation in two consecutive precordial leads; note that acute myocardial infarction may be difficult to rule out in the field). Rule out hypoglycemia in the patient with a history of diabetes (with a fingerstick and glucometer). Rule out a stroke or transient ischemic attack (assessing mental status and administering the Cincinnati Prehospital Stroke Scale). Rule out seizure activity, and rule out an elevated body temperature.
- Determine the patient's serum sodium level because the management of the hyponatremic patient depends on the patient's presentation as well as the serum sodium level. Patients typically fall into one of three groups: mild, moderate, or critical, as described below:
  - Mild hyponatremia (130 to 135 mmol/L) requires observation and restriction of fluids until the patient is able to urinate. Salty foods may be appropriate in small quantities as long as the patient can tolerate them. These patients should be monitored by a health care professional.
    - Reassess the patient every 15 minutes and determine the need for transport to

an emergency department or release of the patient once symptoms have subsided, vital signs are normal, and the serum sodium level is normal. This decision should be made with the consultation of medical control.

- Moderate hyponatremia (124 to 129 mmol/L) requires restriction of fluids given to the patient. The sodium level should be rechecked hourly until the level rises. IV access for a keep-vein-open line should be considered but no fluids administered until the patient is able to urinate. This patient will usually be transported to the emergency department.

- Critical hyponatremia (<124 mmol/L) requires an IV run at a keep-vein-open rate and administration of a diuretic. These patients must be transported to the emergency department as soon as possible. Administration of hypertonic (3%) saline would be an appropriate consideration to help reverse the cerebral edema. Furosemide can be used to overcome the antidiuresis, and the sodium levels should be closely monitored. If the patient is seizing or developing pulmonary or cerebral edema, more urgent and invasive measures must be taken.

Postural Hypotension

Another condition that occurs to athletes at endurance events is the so-called finish-line collapse. This is the development of **postural hypotension**, a drop in the patient's blood pressure when in the upright (erect) standing position. It is also called orthostatic hypotension. A significant difference in the patient's pulse (an increase of 20 points) and systolic blood pressure (a decrease of 20 mm Hg) is generally assumed to be due to hypovolemia or dehydration. In the case of the runner, the hypotension is most likely due to the low peripheral vascular resistance after completing the run. This is further complicated by the sudden stopping of the muscular contractions of the legs, which has been helping aid blood in returning to the heart.

Simple logic would suggest that dehydration would cause stress during the endurance event when the cardiovascular system is under stress—not at the finish line when the body is beginning to relax. The athletes who collapse during the race therefore would likely have serious medical conditions requiring immediate medical attention (ie,

hyperthermia, stroke, acute myocardial infarction or sudden death, seizure or hypoglycemia, or severe dehydration). Postural hypotension has not been proven to be due to dehydration, so the management is no longer aggressive IV fluid therapy.

The management concerns for postural hypotension include:

- If the patient is dizzy or lightheaded, or has a syncopal episode, place the patient in the Trendelenberg position.
- Conduct an initial assessment (assess mental status, airway, breathing, and circulation, and determine priority). Manage the patient's ABCs as you locate any life-threats.
- Obtain a set of baseline vital signs (pulse, respiration, blood pressure, body temperature, and weight).
- Rule out (assess and manage as authorized) ischemic (cardiac) chest pain (ECG and MONA [morphine, oxygen, nitroglycerin, and aspirin], keeping in mind that nitrates are contraindicated in hypotension), lethal dysrhythmias (antidysrhythmics, defibrillation/cardioversion, external pacing), hypoglycemia in patients with diabetes (fingerstick and glucometer), stroke or transient ischemic attack (Cincinnati Prehospital Stroke Scale, computed tomography, and fibrinolytics within 3 hours of symptom onset if embolic stroke), seizure (valium if status epilepticus), and hyperthermia.
- If the patient's serial vital signs do not improve in the Trendelenberg position in 10 to 15 minutes, determine the patient's serum sodium level to rule out hyponatremia.

Acid-Base Balance

The **pH** is a measurement of the hydrogen ion concentration. The normal pH range is 7.35 to 7.45 (▶ **Figure 4-16**). A blood pH greater than 7.45 is called **alkalosis**, and a blood pH of less than 7.35 is called **acidosis**. The mathematical formula for calculating pH is: $pH = -\log [H^+]$. Log refers to the base 10 logarithm and $[H^+]$ refers to the hydrogen ion concentration. Changes in the pH are exponential, not linear. Thus, a change in the pH from 7.40 to 7.20 results in a 10^2 or 100-fold change in the acid concentration.

Normal body functions depend on an acid-base balance that is regulated within a normal physiologic pH range from 7.35 to 7.45. To maintain this delicate balance, the body has buffer systems.

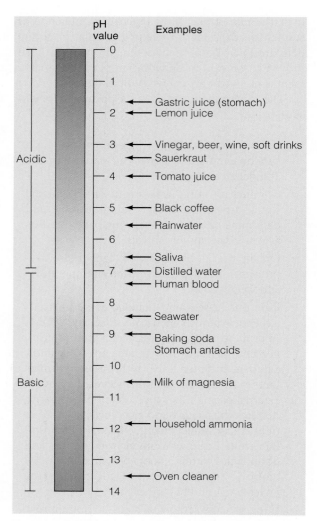

Figure 4-16 The pH scale.

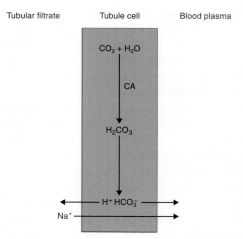

Figure 4-17 Formation and excretion of hydrogen ions by renal tubular epithelial cells in exchange for sodium. CA indicates carbonic anhydrase.

Buffers are molecules that modulate changes in pH to keep it in the physiologic range. In the absence of buffers, the addition of acid to a solution will cause a sharp change in pH. In the presence of a buffer, the pH change will be moderated or may even be unnoticeable. Because acid production is the major challenge to pH homeostasis, most physiologic buffers combine with H^+.

Buffer systems include proteins, phosphate ions, and bicarbonate (HCO_3^-). The large amounts of bicarbonate produced from carbon dioxide (CO_2) made during metabolism create the most important extracellular buffer system of the body (▶ **Figure 4-17**). Hydrogen and bicarbonate ions combine to form carbonic acid (H_2CO_3), which readily dissociates into water and CO_2:

$$H + HCO_3^- \Leftrightarrow H_2CO_3 \Leftrightarrow H_2O + CO_2$$

In the bicarbonate buffer system, excess acid (H^+) combines with bicarbonate (HCO_3^-), forming H_2CO_3. This rapidly dissociates into water and CO_2, which is exhaled. Because the acid is eliminated as water and CO_2, the total pH does not change significantly. A similar process occurs with the production of metabolic base (bicarbonate).

Acid-Base Imbalance

When the buffering capacity of the body is exceeded, acid-base imbalances occur. If the pH is too low (acidosis), neurons become less excitable and central nervous system depression results. Patients become confused and disoriented. If central nervous system depression progresses, the respiratory centers cease to function, causing death.

If pH is too high (alkalosis), neurons become hyperexcitable, firing action potentials at the slightest signal. This condition shows up first as sensory changes, such as numbness or tingling, then as muscle twitches. If alkalosis is severe, muscle twitches turn into sustained contractions (tetanus) that paralyze respiratory muscles.

Disturbances of acid-base balance are associated with disturbances in potassium balance. This is partly due to a kidney transporter that moves H^+ and potassium (K^+) in opposite directions. In acidosis, the kidneys excrete H^+ and resorb K^+. Conversely, when the body goes into a state of alkalosis, the kidneys resorb H^+ and excrete K^+. Potassium imbalance usually shows up as disturbances in excitable tissues, especially the heart.

Acid-base disturbances are classified into two general categories, metabolic and respiratory. Each is then broken down into acidosis and alkalosis. Typi-

Table 4-2
Comparison of Common Acid-Base Disturbances

Disturbance	Primary Abnormality	Compensation	Usual Causes
Metabolic acidosis	Excess endogenous acid depletes bicarbonate	Hyperventilation lowers PCO_2; kidney excretes more hydrogen ions and forms more bicarbonate	Renal failure; ketosis; overproduction of lactic acid
Respiratory acidosis	Inefficient excretion of carbon dioxide by lungs	Formation of additional bicarbonate by kidneys	Chronic pulmonary disease
Metabolic alkalosis	Excess plasma bicarbonate	None	Loss of gastric juice; chloride depletion; excess cortico-steroid hormones; ingestion of excessive bicarbonate or other antacids
Respiratory alkalosis	Hyperventilation lowers PCO_2	Increased excretion	

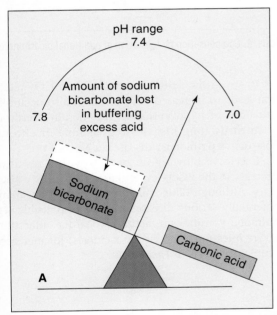
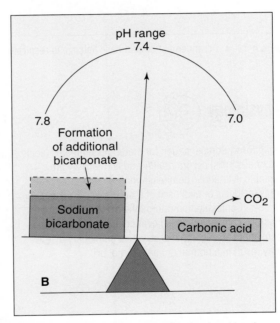

Figure 4-18 A. Derangement of acid-base balance in metabolic acidosis. **B.** Compensation by reduction of carbonic acid and formation of additional bicarbonate.

cal problems that may occur to the patient are shown in ▲ Table 4-2.

<u>Metabolic acidosis</u> is an accumulation of abnormal acids in the blood for any of several reasons (eg, sepsis, diabetic ketoacidosis, and salicylate poisoning). Initially, the partial pressure of carbon dioxide (PCO_2) is not affected, but the pH is decreased. Later, the body compensates for the metabolic abnormality by hyperventilating, leading to excretion of CO_2 and a compensatory respiratory alkalosis. This is why patients with diabetic ketoacidosis often have Kussmaul respirations (deep, rapid sighing ventilations). They are hyperventilating to "blow off" CO_2 and decrease the acidosis (▲ Figure 4-18).

<u>Metabolic alkalosis</u> is a less common condition in acute care, yet very common in chronically ill patients, especially those undergoing nasogastric suction. There is either a build-up of excess metabolic base (eg, chronic antacid ingestion) or a loss of normal acid (eg, through vomiting or nasogastric suctioning). The pH is high and the PCO_2 unchanged initially. Chronically, the body compensates by slowing ventilation and increasing the PCO_2, creating a compensatory respiratory acidosis.

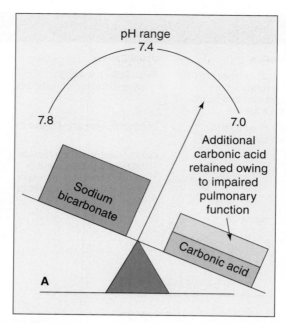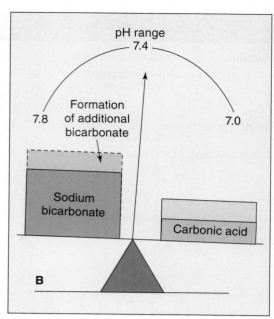

Figure 4-19 A. Derangement of acid-base balance in respiratory acidosis. **B.** Compensation by formation of additional bicarbonate.

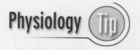

Physiology Tip

Respiratory compensation for metabolic problems (acidosis or alkalosis) occurs *rapidly* and is relatively predictable. Metabolic compensation for respiratory problems (acidosis or alkalosis), if it occurs *at all,* takes hours to days. Compensation returns the pH toward normal. Acutely, compensation is never complete. Chronic compensation, as in chronic obstructive pulmonary disease, may result in a normal or near normal pH.

<u>**Respiratory acidosis**</u> occurs when CO_2 retention leads to increased Pco_2 levels. It also occurs in situations of hypoventilation (eg, heroin overdose) or intrinsic lung diseases (eg, asthma or chronic obstructive pulmonary disease) (▲ **Figure 4-19**).

Excessive blowing off of CO_2 with a resulting decrease in the PCO_2 levels causes <u>**respiratory alkalosis**</u>. Although often called hyperventilation, many potentially serious diseases may be responsible (eg, pulmonary embolism, acute myocardial infarction, severe infection, diabetic ketoacidosis) for increased ventilatory levels (▶ **Figure 4-20**).

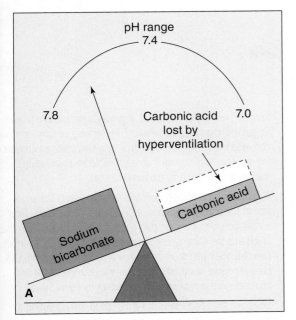 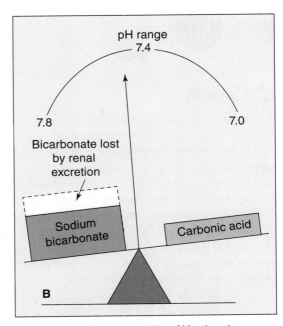

Figure 4-20 **A.** Derangement of acid-base balance in respiratory alkalosis. **B.** Compensation by excretion of bicarbonate.

Physiology Tip

The best treatment for most acid-base disorders is effective treatment of their underlying cause. Always assume that any hyperventilating patient has a potentially serious underlying medical condition. *Never* use the "brown paper bag" approach. Treating patients in this manner can result in hypoxia within 30 seconds.

Case Study

Case Study, Part 4

Completion of Case Study

While en route to the hospital, you consider that older persons are prone to problems with heat because they lose their ability to internally regulate their body temperature. Also, when people get tired, they may not exercise appropriate judgment in potentially dangerous environmental situations, such as staying out in the heat too long. Medications may predispose some people to environmental injury, especially heat illness. Many common medications have anticholinergic side effects, and the result is an impaired ability to sweat and dissipate heat. Heat intolerance is a common side effect of these drugs.

CASE STUDY

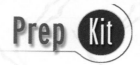

Chapter Summary

- The cellular environment refers to the distribution of cells, molecules, and fluids throughout the body. About 50% to 70% of body weight is fluid (total body water).

- Most of the body's fluid is in the intracellular fluid. The remainder lies outside the cells in the extracellular fluid. Extracellular fluid is further broken down into the interstitial fluid, intravascular fluid, lymph, and transcellular fluid.

- The majority of water is taken in by eating and drinking. A small amount is the product of metabolic reactions. Most water is lost in the urine. The remainder is lost through the skin and lungs, in the feces, and in the sweat.

- Water and dissolved solutes move about via either passive transport (diffusion, facilitated diffusion, osmosis, filtration) or active transport (use of an energy-requiring "carrier pump"). Water moves between intracellular and extracellular fluid by osmosis. It moves from regions of low osmotic pressure to those of higher osmotic pressure. The intracellular fluid volume is controlled by the large amount of proteins and organic compounds that cannot escape through the cell membrane and by the sodium-potassium (Na^+/K^+) membrane pump.

- Water moves between plasma and interstitial fluid based on conditions known as Starling's law. This equilibrium state between the capillary and interstitial space is controlled by capillary hydrostatic pressure, capillary colloidal osmotic pressure, tissue hydrostatic pressure, and tissue colloidal osmotic pressure.

- Edema is the accumulation of excess fluid in the interstitial space. Depending on the cause, edema may be localized (eg, to a single extremity) or generalized (eg, lungs [acute pulmonary edema] and abdomen [ascites]).

- The body's state of hydration is monitored constantly by osmoreceptors, volume-sensitive receptors, and baroreceptors. When osmolarity increases, the pituitary gland releases antidiuretic hormone (ADH). ADH stimulates the kidneys to absorb water, decreasing the osmolarity of the blood. The most potent stimulation for the release of ADH is an increase in blood osmolarity. Changes in blood volume and blood pressure are less of a stimulus.

- Sodium is the most important cation in the body. Most sodium is localized in the extracellular fluid. Normally, only about 10% of the sodium is lost through the skin and gastrointestinal tract. However, sodium loss due to diarrhea, vomiting, extensive burns, or fistula drainage can be considerable. Sweat loss increases greatly with vigorous exercise and exposure to a hot environment.

- Sodium is regulated primarily by the renin-angiotensin-aldosterone system and by hormones called natriuretic pro-

teins. When renin is released, it converts the plasma protein angiotensinogen to angiotensin I. In the lung, angiotensin I is converted rapidly to angiotensin II by an angiotensin converting enzyme. Angiotensin II is responsible for stimulating sodium reabsorption by the renal tubules.

- Angiotensin II is also responsible for stimulating the secretion of the adrenal hormone, aldosterone. Aldosterone acts on the kidney to increase the reabsorption of sodium into the blood and the elimination of potassium in the urine. To maintain balance when there is too much sodium and water, the body produces natriuretic proteins, which inhibit ADH and promote excretion of sodium and water by the kidneys.

- Solutions that body cells are exposed to are classified as isotonic, hypotonic, or hypertonic. Cells that are placed in an isotonic solution, which has the same osmolarity as intracellular fluid (280 mOsm/L), neither shrink nor swell. When cells are placed in a hypertonic solution (has a greater osmolarity than intracellular fluid), they shrink as the water is pulled out of the cell. When cells are placed in a hypotonic solution (has a lower osmolarity than intracellular fluid), they swell.

- Hypernatremia is defined as a serum sodium level above 148 mEq/L and a serum osmolarity greater than 295 mOsm/kg. Manifestations depend on the serum sodium level.

- Hyponatremia is defined as a serum sodium level below 135 mEq/L and a serum osmolarity less than 280 mOsm/kg. Causes of either hypernatremia or hyponatremia may include excess sweating from hot environmental conditions or exercise, or gastrointestinal losses through vomiting, diarrhea, inappropriate IV fluids, or diuretics. Manifestations typically depend not only on the absolute sodium level, but also the time period during which the abnormality developed.

- Potassium is the major intracellular cation and is critical to many functions of the cell. Potassium (K^+) levels may be normal, low (hypokalemia), or elevated (hyperkalemia).

- Calcium enters the body through the gastrointestinal tract and is absorbed from the intestine in a vitamin D–dependent process. It is then stored in the bone and ultimately excreted by the kidney. Calcium levels may be normal, low (hypocalcemia), or elevated (hypercalcemia).

- Phosphate is primarily an intracellular anion and is essential to many body functions. Phosphate levels may be normal, low (hypophosphatemia), or elevated (hyperphosphatemia).

- Magnesium is the second most abundant intracellular cation. Serum levels may be normal, low (hypomagnesemia), or high (hypermagnesemia).

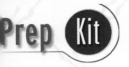

Vital Vocabulary

acidosis A condition in which blood pH is lower than 7.35.

active transport Movement of particles across membranes requiring energy for the movement from an area of low concentration to an area of high concentration.

aldosterone A hormone secreted by the adrenal gland that acts on the kidney to increase resorption of sodium into the blood and elimination of potassium in the urine.

alkalosis A condition in which the blood pH is greater than 7.45.

angiotensin II The chemical responsible for stimulating sodium resorption by the kidneys, decreasing blood flow to the kidneys, and decreasing the glomerular filtration rate.

antidiuretic hormone (ADH) A hormone involved in the water balance of the body.

ascites An abnormal accumulation of fluid in the peritoneal cavity.

baroreceptors Receptors found in the carotid sinus and aortic arch that sense changes in the patient's blood pressure.

buffers Molecules that modulate changes in pH to keep it in the physiologic range.

cellular environment The distribution of cells, molecules, and fluids throughout the body.

edema Accumulation of excess fluid in the interstitial space.

extracellular fluid Fluid found outside of the cells but within the body.

hypercalcemia An increased serum calcium level.

hyperkalemia An elevated blood serum potassium level.

hypermagnesemia An increased serum magnesium level.

hypernatremia A blood serum sodium level greater than 148 mEq/L and a serum osmolarity greater than 295 mOsm/kg.

hyperphosphatemia An elevated blood serum phosphate level.

hypertonic solution A solution with an osmolarity greater than the intracellular fluid.

hypocalcemia A decreased serum calcium level.

hypokalemia A decreased blood serum potassium level.

hypomagnesemia A decreased serum magnesium level.

hyponatremia A blood serum sodium level that is below 135 mEq/L and a serum osmolarity that is less than 280 mOsm/kg.

hypophosphatemia A decreased blood serum phosphate level.

hypotonic solution A solution with an osmolarity lower than the intracellular fluid.

interstitial fluid The fluid found between the cells.

intracellular fluid The fluid found within the cells of the body.

intravascular fluid The fluid found within the blood vessels.

isotonic solution A solution with the same osmolarity as intracellular fluid (280 mOsm/L).

metabolic acidosis An accumulation of abnormal acids in the blood for any of several reasons causing the patient's blood pH to be less than 7.35.

metabolic alkalosis A condition in which the patient's blood pH is greater than 7.45.

natriuretic proteins A protein that increases the rate of excretion of sodium in the urine.

osmoreceptors Sensory receptors located primarily in the hypothalamus that monitor extracellular osmolarity.

osmosis The movement of a solvent, such as water, from an area of low solute concentration to one of high concentration through a selectively permeable membrane to equalize concentrations of a solute on both sides of the membrane.

osmotic pressure The pressure that develops when two solutions of different concentrations are separated by a semipermeable membrane.

passive transport The movement of particles or fluids across membranes without energy through the mechanism of diffusion, facilitated diffusion, osmosis, or filtration.

pH A measure of the concentration of the hydrogen ions with a normal blood range between 7.35 and 7.45.

pitting edema Edema that manifests as tissue in which a temporary "pit" is created by compression with a finger.

postural hypotension A drop in a patient's blood pressure when in the upright (erect) standing position.

renin-angiotensin-aldosterone system (RAAS) A complex feedback mechanism responsible for the kidney's regulation of sodium in the body.

respiratory acidosis A condition that occurs when CO_2 retention leads to increased PCO_2 levels. The patient's blood pH is less than 7.35.

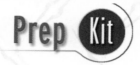

respiratory alkalosis Excessive "blowing off" of CO_2 with a resulting decrease in the PCO_2 causing the blood pH to be greater than 7.45.

solutes Molecules that are dissolved in water.

Starling's law The equilibrium state between the capillary and interstitial space, as first described by E.H. Starling, which is controlled by the efforts of the opposing forces of capillary hydrostatic pressure, capillary colloidal pressure, tissue hydrostatic pressure, and the tissue colloidal osmotic pressure.

tonicity The tension exerted on cell size due to water movement across a cell membrane.

total body water The amount of water found in all parts of the body combined, which is about 50% to 70% of the total body weight.

transcellular fluid The following fluids: cerebrospinal fluid, aqueous and vitreous humors in the eyes, synovial fluid in joints, serous fluid in body cavities (eg, pleural fluid), and glandular secretion fluid.

volume-sensitive receptors Receptors located in the atria that respond to stretch.

Case Study Answers

Question 1: What are the typical ways the body loses water, and how much water can be lost through sweating?

Answer: Most of the body's water is lost in urine (60%). The remainder is lost through the skin and lungs (28%), feces (6%), and sweat (6%). In hot environmental conditions or during periods of rigorous exercise, the amount of water lost through sweating is highly variable. Vomiting and diarrhea can also result in large amounts of fluid loss.

Question 2: What causes a hypotonic fluid deficit, and what are the signs and symptoms associated with it?

Answer: A hypotonic fluid deficit is caused by excessive sodium loss or hyponatremia. Hyponatremia can occur with excess sweating in hot environments or during exercise, or gastrointestinal losses through vomiting, diarrhea, or diuresis. Signs and symptoms of hyponatremia include altered mental status, either mild to severe, headache, depression, weakness, anorexia, nausea, vomiting, abdominal cramps, diarrhea, and pitting edema.

Question 3: How does the body monitor water balance?

Answer: The body monitors its state of hydration with special receptors located in the brain, blood vessels, and kidneys. When osmoreceptors sense an increase in osmolarity, the pituitary gland releases a hormone to stimulate the kidney to resorb water. Volume-sensitive receptors release natriuretic proteins, and baroreceptors sense changes in blood pressure.

Question 4: How can diuretic therapy (water pills) affect the body's electrolyte balance?

Answer: Diuretic therapy, if not carefully monitored, can decrease the sodium, potassium, calcium, and magnesium levels and alter the acid-base balance. The effects include altered mental status, weakness, muscle cramps, cardiac dysrhythmias, and convulsions. It is not uncommon for a patient receiving diuretic therapy to take prescription potassium to help balance the loss of potassium caused by diuretics.

Question 5: What type of solution is normal saline classified as: isotonic, hypotonic, or hypertonic? Why is the solution a first choice for use in the management of dehydration?

Answer: Normal saline is an electrolyte solution of sodium chloride in water and it is isotonic with the extracellular fluid. An isotonic solution such as normal saline is a great choice for dehydration because it causes an immediate expansion of the circulatory volume and it has the same osmolarity as intracellular fluid.

Question 6: How does water move between intracellular fluid and extracellular fluid?

Answer: Osmosis is the movement of water down its concentration gradient across a membrane. This is how water moves between intracellular and extracellular fluid.

Question 7: What protein and what type of pressure are responsible for causing edema in the lower extremities of this patient?

Answer: The protein albumin is responsible for maintaining osmotic pressure, which directly affects the movement of fluid (mostly water) from the tissues back into the blood. When there is a decreased production of albumin from the liver, the osmotic pressure is reduced and fluid leaks into the tissues, causing edema. As paramedics in the field, we often treat patients who have edema. The key is to begin to distinguish between systemic edema, such as that found in the patient with chronic heart failure, and edema in the lungs that can be life-threatening and will need to be managed in the field.

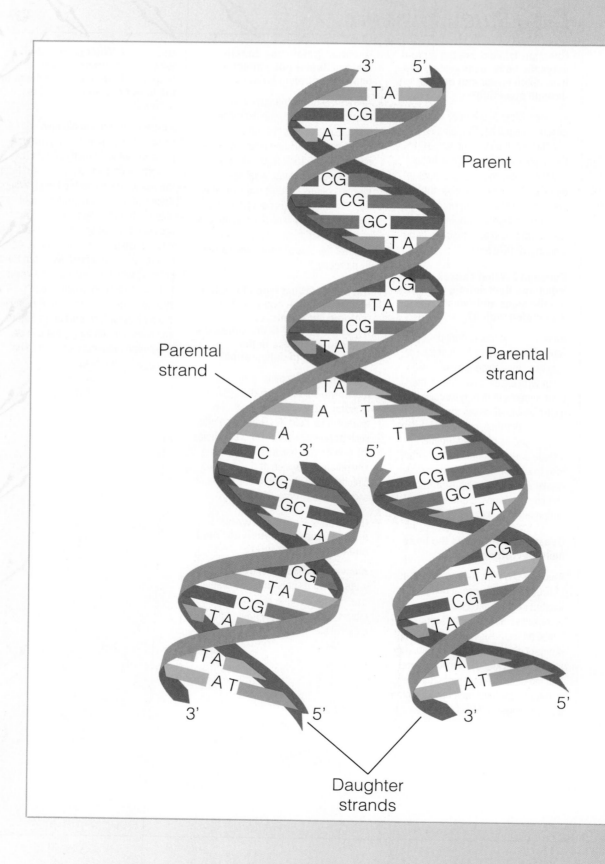

3' 5'

T A
C G
A T

Parent

C G
C G
G C
T A

C G
T A
C G
T A

Parental
strand

Parental
strand

T A
A   T
A   T
A   G
C   3'   5'   C G
C G   G C
G C   T A
T A
C G   C G
T A   T A
C G   C G
T A   T A

T A   T A
A T   A T
3'   5'   3'   5'

Daughter
strands

Genetics and Familial Diseases

5

OBJECTIVES

Cognitive

1-6.5 Discuss analyzing disease risk. (p 73)

1-6.6 Describe environmental risk factors. (p 72)

1-6.7 Discuss combined effects and interaction among risk factors. (p 72–73)

1-6.8 Describe aging as a risk factor for disease. (p 72)

1-6.9 Discuss familial diseases and associated risk factors. (p 73–74)

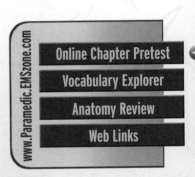

www.Paramedic.EMSzone.com

TECHNOLOGY

Online Chapter Pretest

Vocabulary Explorer

Anatomy Review

Web Links

Chapter FEATURES

Case Studies

Physiology Tips

Medication Tips

Paramedic Safety Tips

Special Needs Tips

Vital Vocabulary

Prep Kit

Factors Causing Disease

Genetic, environmental, age-related, and sex-associated factors can all cause disease. Genetic factors are present at birth and are passed on through a person's genes to future generations. Environmental factors include microorganisms, immunologic and toxic exposures, personal habits and lifestyle, exposures to chemicals, the physical environment, and the psychosocial environment.

Age and sex-associated factors interact with a combination of genetic and environmental factors, lifestyle, and anatomic or hormonal differences. The risk of a particular disease often depends on the patient's age. For example, newborns are at greater risk of certain diseases because their immune systems are not fully developed. Teenagers are at high risk of other diseases due to trauma, drugs, and alcohol. The older we become, the greater the risk of cancer, heart disease, stroke, and Alzheimer's disease.

Some diseases are more prevalent in men, such as lung cancer, gout, and Parkinson's disease. Women are more likely to have osteoporosis, rheumatoid arthritis, and breast cancer. There are uncontrollable factors (eg, genetics) that influence a disease process, but there are also many that can be controlled.

Individuals have control over their lifestyles. Behaviors such as smoking, drinking alcohol, poor nutrition (eg, excessive fat, salt, and sugar intake; insufficient intake of protein, fruits, vegetables, and fiber), lack of exercise, and stress can be modified to improve a person's quality of life. A comprehensive set of disease prevention and health promotion objectives for the nation was published by the US Department of Health and Human Services in the document *Healthy People 2010* (▼ **Figure 5-1**). The

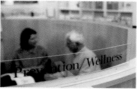
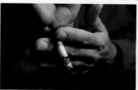
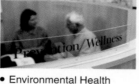
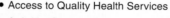
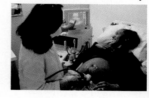
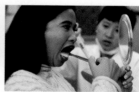
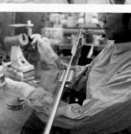
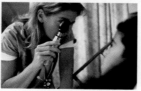

- Access to Quality Health Services
- Arthritis, Osteoporosis, and Chronic Back Conditions
- Cancer
- Chronic Kidney Disease
- Disability and Secondary Conditions
- Educational and Community-Based Programs
- Environmental Health
- Family Planning
- Food Safety
- Health Communication
- Heart Disease and Stroke
- HIV
- Immunization and Infectious Diseases
- Injury and Violence Prevention
- Maternal, Infant, and Child Health
- Medical Product Safety
- Mental Health and Mental Disorders
- Nutrition and Obesity
- Occupational Health and Safety
- Oral Health
- Physical Activity and Fitness
- Public Health Infrastructure
- Respiratory Diseases
- Sexually Transmitted Diseases
- Substance Abuse
- Tobacco Use
- Vision and Hearing

Figure 5-1 *Healthy People 2010* is a comprehensive set of disease prevention and health promotion objectives for Americans to achieve over the first decade of the new century. Specific objectives in each of these 27 focus areas support the overarching objectives of increasing quality and years of healthy life and eliminating health disparities.

Physiology Tip

<u>Autosomal dominant</u> is a pattern of inheritance that involves genes that are located on autosomes (any chromosome other than sex chromosomes). In autosomal dominant inheritance, a person only needs to inherit one copy of a particular form of a gene in order to show that trait. It does not matter what form of the gene is inherited from the other parent. A parent has at least a 50% chance of passing on an autosomal dominant inherited condition to his or her child. One example of an autosomal dominant pattern of inheritance occurs in familial adenomatous polyposis (FAP), which places people at extremely high risk for the development of colon cancer. If a person inherits a copy of the FAP gene from only one parent, there is an increased risk for colon cancer.

dietary and nondietary risk factors that contribute to chronic disease are illustrated in ▶ **Figure 5-2**.

Analyzing Disease Risk

Analyzing disease risk involves consideration of disease rates and disease risk factors (both causal and noncausal). ▶ **Figure 5-3** illustrates methods for analyzing data associated with a disease. Studies of disease should consider, at a minimum, the incidence, prevalence, and mortality of each specific disease. These key terms are described below:

- <u>Incidence</u> is the frequency of disease occurrence (eg, one in four patients has this disease).
- <u>Prevalence</u> is the number of cases in a particular population over time (eg, last year, more than 100,000 patients had this disease).
- <u>Mortality</u> is the number of deaths from a disease in a given population (eg, 1 in 50 affected individuals in the United States with this disease will die).

There is typically interaction among risk factors, age, and sex differences. For example, a person may have a genetic tendency toward coronary artery disease. The risk of a myocardial infarction or sudden death is higher in such an individual even if he or she exercises regularly and has no other risk factors. On the other hand, a person who smokes heavily but has no other risk factors may be at a similarly elevated risk.

Case Study

Case Study, Part 1

Your unit is dispatched to a residence for a 46-year-old man with abdominal pain. The residence is in an upscale neighborhood and, after establishing the scene is safe, you are welcomed into the living room. You find a thin man reclining in a chair. He appears pale, jaundiced, and moderately to severely distressed. A visiting nurse explains that the patient has liver cancer and today he needs transport to the hospital for evaluation of his progressively worsening abdominal pain.

Your general impression is that the patient is middle-aged and terminally ill. He has an IV pump running with pain medication. He is conscious and alert but distracted by his pain. He allows you to obtain his vital signs and is able to answer your questions.

You find out from the nurse that the cancer is progressing rapidly and that the patient also has type 2 diabetes, hepatitis C, and an iron disorder called hemochromatosis. The hospital is expecting the patient for a direct admission.

Initial Assessment

Recording time
2 minutes

Appearance
Moderate to severely distressed

Level of consciousness
Alert

Airway
Open

Vital Signs

Pulse rate/quality
88 beats/min and regular

Blood pressure
160/90 mm Hg

Respiratory rate/depth
20 breaths/min, nonlabored

Question 1: What are the causes of cancer?

Question 2: Are all of the patient's medical problems related to cancer?

Question 3: How is hemochromatosis passed from one generation to the next?

CASE STUDY

Common Familial Diseases and Associated Risk Factors

The terms genetic risk and familial tendency are often used interchangeably. A true genetic risk is one that is passed through generations on a gene. This is not always the case for a familial tendency. Rather, familial diseases may "cluster" in family groups despite lack of evidence for heritable gene-associated abnormalities. Below, we discuss common conditions that often demonstrate a familial tendency. When specific genetic tendencies are

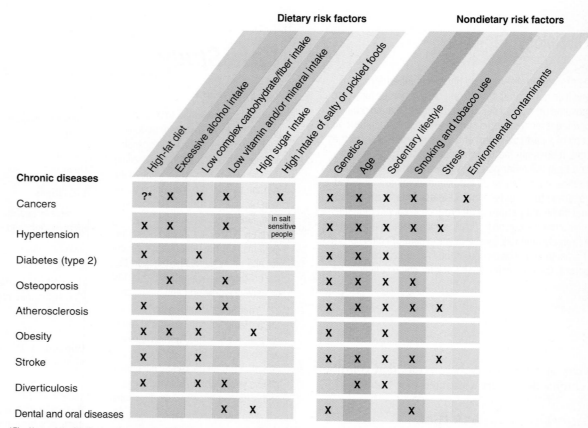

Figure 5-2 Risk factors for chronic diseases. Diet, lifestyle choices, and genetics interact to shape a person's risk profile.

Chronic diseases	High-fat diet	Excessive alcohol intake	Low complex carbohydrate/fiber intake	Low vitamin and/or mineral intake	High sugar intake	High intake of salty or pickled foods	Genetics	Age	Sedentary lifestyle	Smoking and tobacco use	Stress	Environmental contaminants
Cancers	?*	X	X	X		X	X	X	X	X		X
Hypertension	X	X		X		in salt sensitive people	X	X	X	X	X	
Diabetes (type 2)	X		X				X	X	X			
Osteoporosis		X		X			X	X	X	X		
Atherosclerosis	X		X	X			X	X	X	X	X	
Obesity	X	X	X		X		X		X			
Stroke	X		X				X	X	X	X	X	
Diverticulosis	X		X	X				X	X			
Dental and oral diseases			X	X			X			X		

*The Nurses' Health Study, a large prospective study, found no evidence linking higher total fat intake with increased risk of breast cancer. These results call into question theories that link dietary fat to other cancers.

known, they will be noted and discussed. Examples of traits and diseases carried on human chromosomes are described in ▶ **Table 5-1**.

<u>**Autosomal recessive**</u> is another pattern of inheritance that involves genes located on autosomes. In autosomal recessive inheritance, a person needs to inherit two copies of a particular form of a gene in order to show that trait. A parent who carries the gene for an autosomal recessive trait but does not display the trait has a 25% chance of passing the inherited condition to his or her child if the other parent is also a carrier for the trait. If both parents actually have the inherited condition, then all children will also have the condition. One example of an autosomal recessive pattern of inheritance occurs in hemochromatosis, which causes people to accumulate too much iron in their bodies. A person must inherit a copy of the hemochromatosis gene from each parent in order to develop the disease.

Immunologic Disorders

Immunologic diseases are caused by either hyperactivity or hypoactivity of the immune system (see Chapter 7, Self-Defense Mechanisms). Most immunologic diseases that exhibit familial tendencies involve an overactive immune system. Specific examples include allergies, asthma, and rheumatic fever.

- Allergies are acquired following initial exposure to a stimulant, known as an <u>**allergen**</u>. Repeated exposures cause a reaction by the immune system to the allergen (▶ **Figure 5-4**). Clinical presentation varies but usually includes swelling and itching, runny nose, coughing, sneezing, wheezing, and nasal congestion. The medical term for having an allergic tendency is <u>**atopic**</u>. In addition to the genetic predisposition for atopy and its associated conditions, environmental interactions are involved. Environmental conditions may trigger a shift in susceptibility toward an allergic reaction.

- <u>**Asthma**</u> is a chronic inflammatory condition resulting in intermittent wheezing and excess mucus production. Nearly 60% of attacks are precipitated by viral infections in susceptible

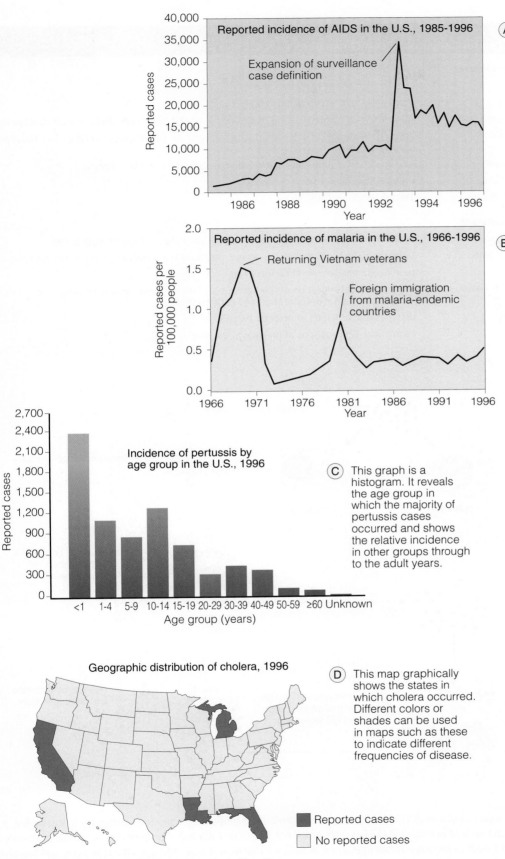

(A) This line graph shows actual number of cases over an extended period of time.

(B) This graph shows the number of cases per 100,000 people. It takes into account the growing population in the United States over the 30-year period. This factor affects the graph considerably.

(C) This graph is a histogram. It reveals the age group in which the majority of pertussis cases occurred and shows the relative incidence in other groups through to the adult years.

(D) This map graphically shows the states in which cholera occurred. Different colors or shades can be used in maps such as these to indicate different frequencies of disease.

Figure 5-3 Four methods for analyzing data associated with a disease.

Table 5-1
Traits and Diseases Carried on Human Chromosomes

Autosomal recessive

Albinism	Lack of pigment in eyes, skin, and hair
Cystic fibrosis	Pancreatic failure, mucus build-up in lungs
Sickle cell anemia	Abnormal hemoglobin leading to sickle-shaped red blood cells that obstruct vital capillaries
Tay-Sachs disease	Improper metabolism of a class of chemicals called gangliosides in nerve cells, resulting in early death
Phenylketonuria	Accumulation of phenylalanine in blood; results in mental retardation
Attached earlobe	Earlobe attached to skin
Hyperextendable thumb	Thumb bends past 45° angle

Autosomal dominant

Achondroplasia	Dwarfism resulting from a defect in epiphyseal plates of forming long bones
Marfan's syndrome	Defect manifested in connective tissue, resulting in excessive growth, aortic rupture
Widow's peak	Hairline coming to a point on forehead
Huntington's disease	Progressive deterioration of the nervous system beginning in late twenties or early thirties; results in mental deterioration and early death
Brachydactyly	Disfiguration of hands, shortened fingers
Freckles	Permanent aggregations of melanin in the skin

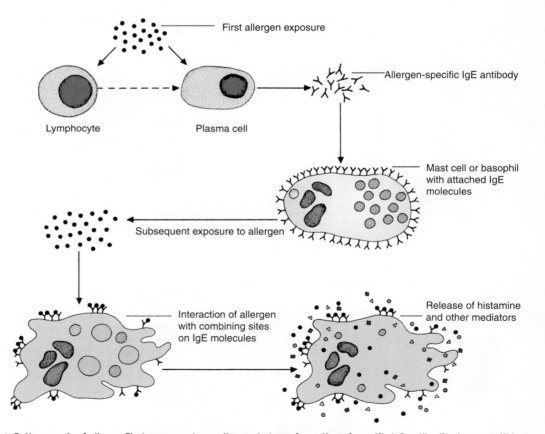

Figure 5-4 Pathogenesis of allergy. First exposure to an allergen induces formation of specific IgE antibodies in susceptible individuals, which then bind to mast cells and basophils by the nonantigen receptor end of the molecule. Subsequent exposure to the same allergen leads to antigen-antibody interaction, liberating histamine and other mediators from mast cells and basophils. These mediators induce allergic manifestations.

individuals. Allergies account for another 20% of cases, with stress and emotions causing the remainder. In addition to a familial component, recent studies have suggested that chromosomal differences in certain individuals result in the susceptibility to asthma. Often there is significant overlap between causative factors, including the patient's environment. There are a number of other common respiratory diseases caused by environmental pollutants, viruses, or bacteria (▶ Table 5-2).

- **Rheumatic fever** is an inflammatory disease that occurs primarily in children. The disease results from a delayed reaction to an untreated streptococcal infection of the upper respiratory tract (eg, strep throat). Symptoms appear several weeks after the acute infection and include fever, abdominal pain, vomiting, arthritis, palpitations, and chest pain. Recurrent episodes of rheumatic fever may cause permanent myocardial damage, especially to the cardiac valves (▶ Figure 5-5). A family history of acute rheumatic fever may predispose an individual to the disease.

Cancer

Cancer includes a large number of malignant growths (neoplasms). The prognosis often depends on the extent of its spread when found, known as *metastasis*, and the effectiveness of treatment.

Lung cancer is the leading cause of death due to cancer in the United States (▶ Table 5-3). The major risk factor is cigarette smoking. Research has identified eight alterations in the genetic material of lung cancers that suggest a genetic tendency. Other predisposing factors include exposure to asbestos, coal products, and other industrial and chemical products. Symptoms include cough, difficulty breathing, blood-tinged sputum, and repeated infections. Treatment depends on the type, site, and extent of the cancer and may include surgery, chemotherapy, and/or radiotherapy.

Breast cancer is the most common type of cancer occurring among women and accounts for as many as 178,700 newly diagnosed cases and 48,000 deaths each year (▶ Figure 5-6). Women whose first-degree relatives (ie, parent, sister, or daughter) have breast cancer are 2.1 times as likely to develop the disease. Risk varies with the age at which the affected relative was diagnosed: the younger the age at occurrence, the greater the risk posed to relatives. Approximately 5% to 10% of patients with breast cancer demonstrate a pattern of autosomal dominant inheritance. This is characterized by transmission of cancer predisposition

---

Case Study

Case Study, Part 2

You discover that the patient has been unable to eat today and has lost a significant amount of weight in the last month. The focused physical exam (cardiopulmonary system) reveals lung sounds that are clear and visible jugular vein distention when the patient is seated in the semi-Fowler's position. There is a right upper quadrant mass that is tender to touch. The patient feels warm and dry. You obtain his temperature, which indicates he has a low-grade fever. The SAMPLE history adds the following findings: the patient has no allergies and, except for the pain medication, he has discontinued all other medications and treatments. He is resigned to the fact that he has a short time to live and would like to be made as comfortable as possible. You obtain a blood glucose reading and attach your ECG monitor to the patient. You have also begun treatment by administering oxygen by cannula and are carefully moving him to the ambulance on a stretcher.

Focused Physical Assessment

Recording time
5 minutes

Skin signs
Warm, dry, jaundiced, and pale

Lung sounds
Clear bilaterally
No pedal edema but visible jugular vein distention

Diagnostic Tools

Electrocardiogram
Normal sinus rhythm with no ectopy

SpO₂
98%

Blood glucose level
99 mg/dL (normal range, 80–120 mg/dL)

Question 4: How is the prognosis for cancer determined?

Question 5: Is liver cancer one of the leading causes of death from cancer?

CASE STUDY

Table 5-2
Common Respiratory Diseases

Disease	Symptoms	Cause	Treatment
Emphysema	Breakdown of alveoli; shortness of breath	Smoking and air pollution	Administer oxygen to relieve symptoms; quit smoking; avoid polluted air. No known cure.
Chronic bronchitis	Coughing, shortness of breath	Smoking and air pollution	Quit smoking; move out of polluted area; if possible, move to warmer, drier climate.
Acute bronchitis	Inflammation of the bronchi; yellowy mucus coughed up; shortness of breath	Many viruses and bacteria	If bacterial, take antibiotics, cough medicine; use vaporizer.
Sinusitis	Inflammation of the sinuses; mucus discharge; blockage of nasal passageways; headache	Many viruses and bacteria	If bacterial, take antibiotics and decongestant tablets; use vaporizer.
Laryngitis	Inflammation of larynx and vocal cords; sore throat; hoarseness; mucus build-up and cough	Many viruses and bacteria	If bacterial, take antibiotics, cough medicine; avoid irritants, such as smoke; avoid talking.
Pneumonia	Inflammation of the lungs ranging from mild to severe; cough and fever; shortness of breath at rest; chills; sweating; chest pains; blood in mucus	Bacteria, viruses, or inhalation of irritating gases	Consult physician immediately; go to bed; take antibiotics, cough medicine; stay warm.
Asthma	Constriction of bronchioles; mucus build-up in bronchioles; periodic wheezing; difficulty breathing	Allergy to pollen, some foods, food additives; dandruff from dogs and cats; exercise	Use inhalants to open passageways; avoid irritants.

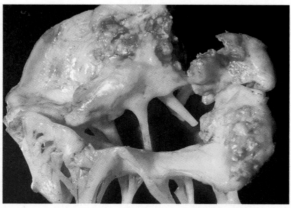

Figure 5-5 Poorly functioning scarred and calcified mitral valve resulting from valve damage caused by rheumatic fever. Valve was excised and replaced with an artificial heart valve.

Table 5-3
Estimated Cancer Deaths in US 2004

Cancer Type	Estimated Deaths
Lung	170,000
Colon/Rectum	55,000
Breast	48,000
Prostate	36,000
Lymphoma	28,000
Leukemia	22,000
Liver	12,000
Skin	10,000
Cervix	5,000
Total (all cancers)	600,000

from generation to generation, with approximately 50% of susceptible individuals inheriting the predisposing genetic alteration. The susceptibility may be inherited through either the mother's or the father's side of the family, as illustrated in the tracking of two breast cancer mutations shown in ▶ **Figure 5-7**.

Early symptoms of breast cancer are usually detected by the woman during breast self-examination and include a small, painless lump, thick or dimpled skin, or a change in the nipple. Later symptoms include nipple discharge, pain, and swollen lymph glands in the axilla. Treatment depends on the location and size of the tumor and whether or not it has spread to other areas (▶ **Figure 5-8**).

Colorectal cancer is the third most common type of cancer in both males and females, accounting for

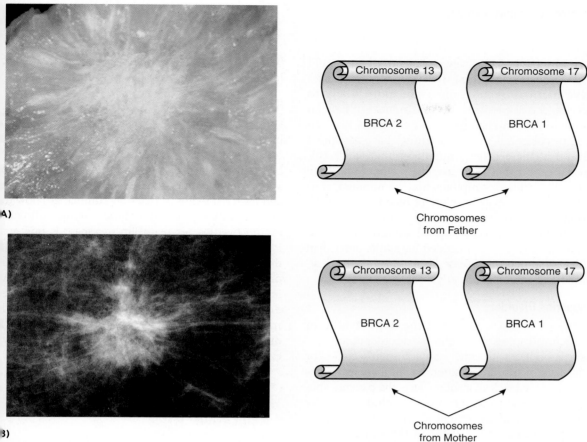

Figure 5-6 Breast carcinoma. **A.** Cross-section of breast biopsy. Tumor appears as firm, poorly circumscribed mass that infiltrates the surrounding fatty breast tissue. **B.** Appearance of breast carcinoma in a mammogram. Tumor appears as a white area with infiltrating margins. Note that the same criteria used to identify breast carcinoma on gross examination are used to recognize malignant neoplasms in the mammogram.

Figure 5-7 Mutations on chromosomes 13 and 17, from either parent, can make a patient more susceptible to breast cancer.

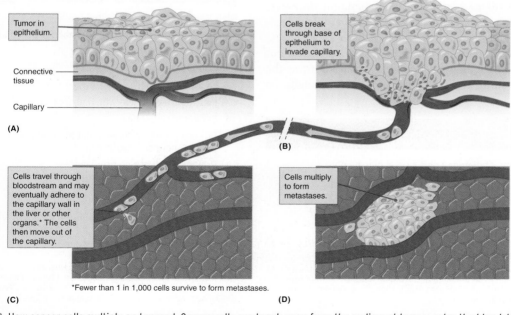

*Fewer than 1 in 1,000 cells survive to form metastases.

Figure 5-8 How cancer cells multiply and spread. Cancer cells can break away from the malignant tumor, enter the bloodstream or lymphatic system, and travel to new sites to form new tumors in other organs.

a combined 131,600 newly diagnosed cases and 55,000 deaths each year. Relatives of people who have had colorectal cancer are more likely to develop the disease themselves. Parents can pass on to their children changes on certain genes that can lead to colorectal cancer. Scientists have identified several of these genetic mutations that cause colorectal cancer, but there are likely others that have yet to be defined. Symptoms may be minimal, consisting only of small amounts of blood in the stool. Treatment involves surgery and sometimes chemotherapy. Periodic rectal examinations and colonoscopy are recommended for adults older than 40 years so that the disease, if present, may be diagnosed and treated at an early stage.

Endocrine Disorders

Diabetes mellitus is one of the most significant endocrine diseases. It is a chronic disorder of metabolism associated with either partial insulin secretion or total lack of insulin secretion by the pancreas. This partial or total lack of insulin affects the patient's ability to utilize glucose. Symptoms include excessive thirst and urination, weight abnormalities, and the presence of excessive sugar in the urine and the blood. The disease is common and evidence suggests that the incidence is increasing. The diagnosis criteria for diabetes are listed in ▼ Table 5-4. There are two major forms: ketoacidosis prone and nonketoacidosis prone. Ketoacidosis prone, or **type 1 diabetes**, is sometimes known as *insulin-dependent diabetes mellitus* because patients need exogenous insulin to survive. Nonketoacidosis prone, or **type 2 diabetes**, may be termed *non-insulin-dependent diabetes,* although many type II diabetics still require exogenous insulin injections to survive. Both forms have a hereditary predisposition. Type 1 diabetes is without a cure (other than pancreas transplantation) at the present time; type 2 diabetes can occasionally be

brought under control with weight loss. The risk factors for diabetes mellitus are shown in ▼ Table 5-5.

Hematologic Disorders

Hemolytic anemia is an anemia that is characterized by increased destruction of red blood cells. This disorder has a number of causes, such as an Rh factor blood transfusion reaction, a disorder of the immune system, or exposure to chemicals, such as benzene and bacterial toxins. ► Figure 5-9 summarizes how the body handles iron. Hemolytic anemia following aspirin overdose or penicillin treatment is rare; it is much more common, although still rare, with sulfa drugs used to treat urinary tract infection (eg, Septra or Bactrim [trimethoprim-sulfamethoxazole]). An inherited enzyme deficiency (glucose-6-phosphatase dehydrogenase [G-6-PD] deficiency) markedly increases a person's susceptibility to sulfa drug–induced hemolytic anemia. ► Table 5-6 shows examples of inherited hemolytic anemias.

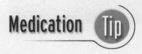

Medication Tip

Drugs are only one of many possible causes of hemolytic anemias.

Table 5-4
Diagnostic Criteria for Diabetes Mellitus

Symptoms of diabetes plus causal plasma glucose concentration ≥200 mg/dL (11.1 mmol/L)

or

Fasting plasma glucose ≥126 mg/dL (7.0 mmol/L)

or

Two-hour plasma glucose ≥200 mg/dL (11.1 mmol/L) during an oral glucose tolerance test

© 2003 American Diabetes Association. Reprinted with permission from American Diabetes Association. From *Diabetes Care* 2003 (suppl 1): S5-S20.

Table 5-5
Risk Factors for Type 1 and Type 2 Diabetes Mellitus

Risk Factors for Type 1 Diabetes
- First-degree relative (parent, sibling) with diabetes

Risk Factors for Type 2 Diabetes
- Age ≥ 45 years
- Overweight (BMI ≥25 kg/m^2)
- First-degree relative with diabetes
- Sedentary lifestyle
- Ethnicity: African American, Latino, Native American, Asian American, Pacific Islander
- Previously identified prediabetes
- History of gestational diabetes
- Hypertension (≥140/90 mm Hg)
- HDL cholesterol level ≥35 mg/dL and/or triglyceride level ≥250 mg/dL
- History of vascular disease

© 2003 American Diabetes Association. Reprinted with permission from American Diabetes Association. From *Diabetes Care* 2003; 26 (suppl 1): S140; and *Diabetes Care* 2003; 26 (suppl 1): S140; and *Diabetes Care* 2003; 26 (suppl 1): S62-S69.

<u>Hemophilia</u> is an inherited disorder characterized by excessive bleeding. It is a sex-linked condition, occurring only in males, passed from asymptomatic mothers to sons. Several forms of the disease occur. In all forms, one of the blood-clotting proteins (usually Factor VIII) necessary for normal blood coagulation is missing or present in abnormally low amounts. Patients experience greater than usual blood loss in dental extractions and following simple injuries. They may also bleed into joints and, rarely, into the brain. Treatment consists of administration of missing blood-clotting factors.

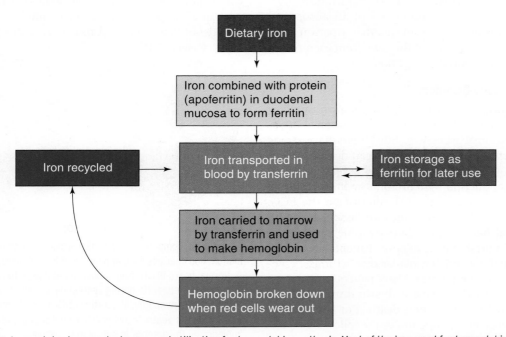

Figure 5-9 Iron uptake, transport, storage, and utilization for hemoglobin synthesis. Most of the iron used for hemoglobin synthesis is recycled from worn-out red cells. Chronic blood loss removes iron-containing cells from the circulation, and the iron contained in the red cells can no longer be recycled to make hemoglobin, which leads to iron deficiency anemia.

Table 5-6
Inheritance and Manifestations of Some Hereditary Hemolytic Anemias

Anemia	Inheritance	Characteristics of Red Cells	Manifestations
Hereditary spherocytosis	Dominant or recessive	Spherocytic	Mild to moderate chronic hemolytic anemia
Hereditary ovalocytosis	Dominant	Oval	Usually asymptomatic; may have mild anemia
Sickle cell anemia	Codominant	Normocytic; cells sickle under reduced oxygen tension	Marked anemia
Hemoglobin C disease	Codominant	Normocytic	Mild to moderate anemia
Thalassemia minor	Dominant (heterozygous)	Hypochromic-microcytic; total number of red cells usually increased	Mild anemia
Thalassemia major	Dominant (homozygous)	Hypochromic-microcytic	Severe anemia; usually fatal in childhood
Glucose-6-phosphatase dehydrogenase deficiency	X-linked recessive	Normocytic; enzyme-deficient cells	Episodes of acute hemolytic anemia precipitated by drugs or infections

<u>Hemochromatosis</u> is an inherited disease in which the body absorbs more iron than it needs. The excess iron is stored in various organs throughout the body, including the liver, kidney, and pancreas. Hemochromatosis can lead to diabetes, heart disease, liver disease, arthritis, impotence, and a bronzed skin color. These symptoms can be avoided by regularly drawing blood (phlebotomy). Hemochromatosis is inherited in an autosomal recessive manner, which means that a person must inherit a mutated copy of the gene from each parent in order to develop the condition.

Cardiovascular Disorders

Several cardiovascular disorders are known to follow specific patterns of inheritance (eg, autosomal dominant, autosomal recessive). Still others have strong familial tendencies (eg, coronary heart disease).

<u>Long QT syndrome</u> is one of several inherited cardiac conduction system abnormalities resulting in a prolongation of the QT interval on the ECG. Sometimes, these syndromes are associated with congenital hearing loss, hypertrophic cardiomyopathy, or mitral valve prolapse. Patients are at risk for palpitations and ventricular dysrhythmias, especially torsades de pointes. Many patients are asymptomatic until they have a dysrhythmia, causing either syncope or sudden death. For this reason, always consider syncope under the following conditions to be due to a life-threatening dysrhythmia until proven otherwise:

- Exercise-induced syncope
- Syncope associated with chest pain
- A history of syncope in a close family member (ie, parent, sibling, or child)
- Syncope associated with startle (eg, loud noises such as phones or alarm clocks)

Because most long QT syndromes are inherited in an autosomal dominant manner, all first-degree relatives must also be screened.

<u>Cardiomyopathy</u> is a general term for disease of the myocardium (heart muscle) that ultimately progresses to heart failure, acute myocardial infarction, or death. These cause the heart muscle to become thin, flabby, dilated, or enlarged. One variant, <u>hypertrophic cardiomyopathy</u>, is hereditary. A comparison in function between the normal heart and the hypertrophic heart is shown in ▶ **Figure 5-10**. The main feature of hypertrophic cardiomyopathy is an excessive thickening of the heart muscle (*hypertrophy* means to thicken or grow excessively). In addition, microscopic examination of the heart muscle in hypertrophic cardiomyopathy shows that it is

abnormal. In the majority of cases the condition is inherited through an autosomal dominant pattern. Thus, in affected families the condition usually passes from one generation to the next and generations are not skipped. Patients may have shortness of breath, chest pains, palpitations, or syncope. Sudden cardiac death is also possible. Medical treatment with beta-blockers is effective in some patients. Others require surgery or an automatic implantable cardiac defibrillator designed to deliver a shock to the heart (▼ **Figure 5-11**).

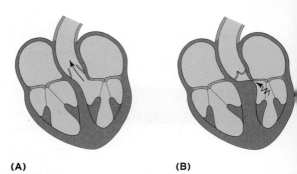

(A)   **(B)**

Figure 5-10 Comparison of normal cardiac function with malfunction characteristic of hypertrophic cardiomyopathy. **A.** Normal heart, illustrating unobstructed flow of blood from left ventricle into aorta during ventricular systole. **B.** Hypertrophic cardiomyopathy, illustrating obstruction to outflow of blood from left ventricle by hypertrophied septum, which impinges on the anterior leaflet of mitral valve.

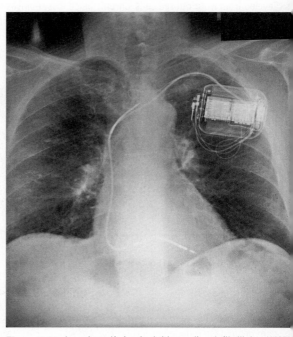

Figure 5-11 An automatic implantable cardiac defibrillator (AICD) is attached directly to the heart and continuously monitors heart rhythm, delivering shocks as needed. The electricity from the AICD is so low that it has no effect on rescuers.

Mitral valve prolapse (MVP) is also referred to as a floppy mitral valve. It is relatively common (2.5% of males, 7.6% of females), and the cause is unknown. The mitral valve leaflets balloon into the left atrium during systole. MVP is often a benign, symptomless condition but may be marked by varied symptoms (eg, chest pain, fatigue, dizziness, dyspnea, or palpitations). Generally, the only physical finding is a "clicking" sound heard during cardiac auscultation. Cardiac arrhythmias develop in a small number of patients. There is a familial tendency toward MVP but usually in association with other cardiovascular conditions.

Sometimes MVP leads to a condition known as mitral regurgitation, or mitral insufficiency, in which a large amount of blood leaks backward through the defective valve. Mitral regurgitation can lead to the thickening or enlargement of the heart wall, caused by the extra pumping the heart must do to make up for the backflow of blood. It sometimes causes people to feel tired or short of breath. Mitral regurgitation usually can be treated with medication, but some people need surgery to repair or replace the defective valve.

Coronary heart disease (often called coronary artery disease) is a disease caused by impaired circulation to the heart. Typically, patients have occluded coronary arteries from atherosclerotic plaque build-up (▼ Figure 5-12). The effects can range from ischemia to infarction and necrosis (death) of the myocardium. Almost half of all cardiovascular deaths result from coronary artery disease. The tendency to develop this condition has been shown to run in families. In addition, a significant risk for coronary artery disease development includes having a father who had an acute myocardial infarction or died suddenly before 55 years of age, or a mother who died before 65 years of age. Other coronary risk factors include:

- **Hypercholesterolemia** – an elevation of the blood cholesterol level. The blood cholesterol

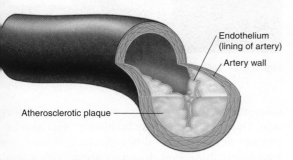

Atherosclerotic plaque

Endothelium (lining of artery)

Artery wall

Figure 5-12 Development of atherosclerosis. Atherosclerosis plaque is formed by a buildup of fatty material in the wall of an artery. An artery narrowed by plaque is vulnerable to blockage by a blood clot, causing a heart attack or stroke.

Case Study

Case Study, Part 3

After the patient has been moved to the ambulance and transport has begun, you perform an ongoing assessment. The patient's symptoms are severe abdominal pain and tenderness, nausea, weakness, and fatigue. His vital signs are relatively unchanged from the baseline set. Although the patient is distressed, he is talkative and does not mind telling you about his medical history. You call the hospital to confirm that a room will be ready and waiting for him upon your arrival.

Ongoing Assessment

Recording time
15 minutes

Symptoms
Severe abdominal pain and tenderness, nausea, weakness, and fatigue

Vital signs
Unchanged from the baseline set

Question 6: What are some of the environmental factors that may have contributed to the development of this patient's cancer?

Question 7: What is type 2 diabetes and is it hereditary?

CASE STUDY

level is further divided into high-density lipoproteins (HDL, or "good cholesterol") and low-density lipoproteins (LDL, or "bad cholesterol"). Despite having a normal total cholesterol level, persons with abnormally low levels of HDL and/or elevations of LDL are still at an increased risk. Adult blood cholesterol levels are listed in ▶ Table 5-7.

- Cigarette smoking – this is a major risk factor closely linked with coronary artery disease and sudden death.
- Hypertension (high blood pressure) – not only is hypertension associated with an increased risk of coronary artery disease, it is also strongly associated with an increased risk of stroke.
- Age – the risk of coronary artery disease increases with men older than 45 years and women older than 55 years.
- Diabetes – both type 1 and type 2 diabetes are associated with increased risk of coronary artery disease and of stroke.

Table 5-7
*Adult Blood Cholesterol and Triglyceride Levels**

Total Cholesterol		LDL Cholesterol	
Desirable	<200	Optimal	<100
Borderline high	200–239	Near optimal/above optimal	100–129
High	≥240	Borderline high	130–159
		High	160–189
		Very high	≥190
Triglyceride		**HDL Cholesterol**	
Normal	<150	Low	<40
Borderline high	150–199	High	≥60
High	200–499		
Very high	≥500		

* All units are in mg/dL.

Reprinted with permission from National Cholesterol Education Program. *Third Report of the Expert Panel on Detection, Evaluation, and Treatment of High Blood Cholesterol in Adults (Adult Treatment Panel III).* Washington, DC: US Department of Health and Human Services; 2001. NIH publication 01-3305.

Renal Disorders

<u>Gout</u> is an abnormal accumulation of uric acid due to a defect in its metabolism. As a result of this defect, uric acid accumulates in the blood and joints, causing pain and swelling of the joints, especially the big toe. Often, the patient also has fever and chills. Uric acid can also accumulate in the kidney, causing kidney stones. Gout is more common among men than women and usually has a genetic basis. If untreated, the disease causes destructive tissue changes in the joints and kidneys. Treatment includes diet and drugs to reduce inflammation and to increase the excretion of uric acid or decrease its formation.

<u>Kidney stones</u> are small masses of uric acid or calcium salts that form in any part of the urinary system (eg, kidney, ureter, or bladder). Often, although not always, stones cause severe pain, nausea, and vomiting when the body attempts to pass them. Although most stones are small, occasionally they increase in size to form structures large enough to adopt the internal contours of the kidney (▶ **Figure 5-13**). Researchers have found a gene that causes the intestines to absorb too much calcium, which can lead to the formation of kidney stones. Uric acid stones often have a genetic basis. Some are small enough to pass in the urine, with or without pain; others must be removed surgically.

Gastrointestinal Disorders

<u>Malabsorption disorders</u> result from defects in the function of the bowel wall that prevent normal absorption of nutrients. The result is a complex of symptoms, including loss of appetite, bloating, weight loss, muscle pain, and stools with high fat

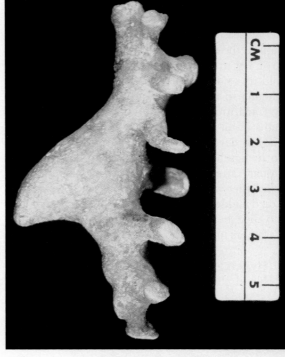

Figure 5-13 Large staghorn-shaped kidney stone.

content, that result from abnormal intestinal absorption. Diarrhea, which may be bloody, may also be a prominent symptom. Although many diseases can lead to malabsorption disorders, those with a familial or genetic component include:

- <u>Lactose intolerance</u> – a defect or deficiency of the enzyme lactase, resulting in an inability to

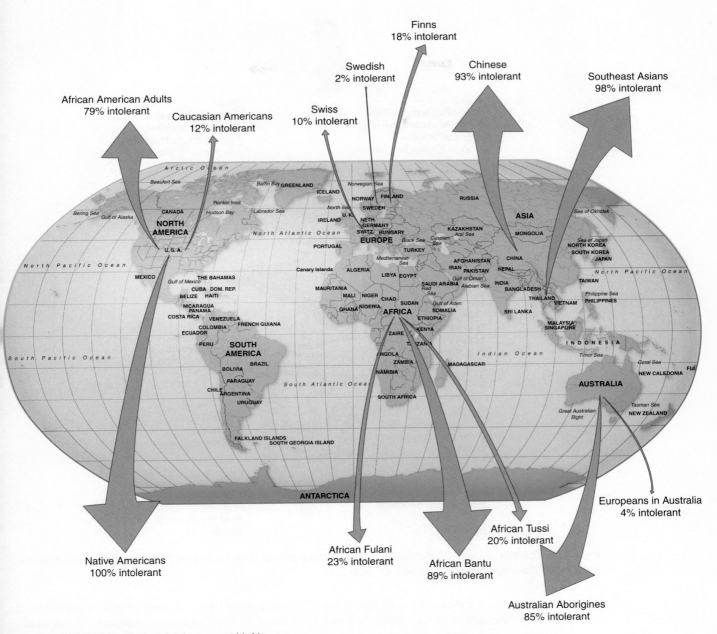

African American Adults
79% intolerant

Caucasian Americans
12% intolerant

Swiss
10% intolerant

Swedish
2% intolerant

Finns
18% intolerant

Chinese
93% intolerant

Southeast Asians
98% intolerant

Native Americans
100% intolerant

African Fulani
23% intolerant

African Bantu
89% intolerant

African Tussi
20% intolerant

Europeans in Australia
4% intolerant

Australian Aborigines
85% intolerant

Figure 5-14 Distribution of lactose intolerance worldwide.

digest lactose (milk sugar). Lactase deficiency affects between 30 and 50 million people in the United States alone. Some estimate that nearly three fourths of the world's population is lactose intolerant (▲ Figure 5-14). Symptoms include bloating, flatulence, abdominal discomfort, nausea, and diarrhea on ingestion of milk and milk products. Lactase deficiency appears to be due to an abnormal gene.

- <u>Ulcerative colitis</u> – a serious chronic inflammatory disease of the large intestine and rectum. It is characterized by recurrent episodes of abdominal pain, fever, chills, and profuse diar-

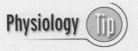

Physiology Tip

Collectively, ulcerative colitis and Crohn's disease are termed inflammatory bowel disease.

rhea, with stools containing pus, blood, and mucus. Treatment consists of anti-inflammatory agents, including corticosteroids. Severe cases may require surgery with removal of parts of

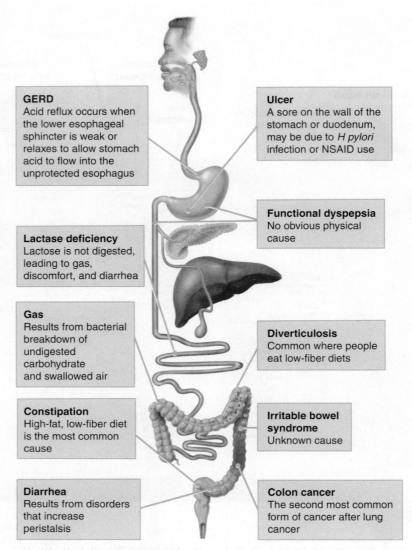

GERD
Acid reflux occurs when the lower esophageal sphincter is weak or relaxes to allow stomach acid to flow into the unprotected esophagus

Ulcer
A sore on the wall of the stomach or duodenum, may be due to *H pylori* infection or NSAID use

Functional dyspepsia
No obvious physical cause

Lactase deficiency
Lactose is not digested, leading to gas, discomfort, and diarrhea

Gas
Results from bacterial breakdown of undigested carbohydrate and swallowed air

Diverticulosis
Common where people eat low-fiber diets

Constipation
High-fat, low-fiber diet is the most common cause

Irritable bowel syndrome
Unknown cause

Diarrhea
Results from disorders that increase peristalsis

Colon cancer
The second most common form of cancer after lung cancer

Figure 5-15 Common gastrointestinal ailments. Beans are familiar culprits in what is perhaps the most common gastrointestinal ailment—gas. Rice is the only starch that does not cause gas.

the intestinal tract. Patients are at increased risk for developing cancer of the colon. Research demonstrates that there is an increased occurrence of ulcerative colitis in families.

- <u>Crohn's disease</u> – a chronic inflammatory condition affecting the colon and/or terminal part of the small intestine. Symptoms include frequent episodes of nonbloody diarrhea, abdominal pain, nausea, fever, weakness, and weight loss. Treatment is by anti-inflammatory agents, antibiotics, and proper nutrition. Although the specific genetic pattern of inheritance has yet to be defined, current research indicates that Crohn's disease is associated with gene abnormalities.

<u>Peptic ulcer disease</u> is characterized by circumscribed erosions in the mucous membrane lining of

the gastrointestinal tract. These ulcerations may occur in the esophagus, stomach, duodenum, or jejunum. The stomach and duodenum are the most common sites. Peptic ulcers may result from excess acid production or from a breakdown in the normal mechanisms protecting the mucous membranes. A major contributor is infection with the bacterium *Helicobacter pylori*. Symptoms include gnawing pain often worse when the stomach is empty, after certain foods have been eaten, or when the patient is under stress. Treatment includes avoidance of irritants (eg, tobacco, alcohol, irritating foods), antibiotics, and drugs to decrease acidity. In refractory cases, surgery may be necessary. The cause of peptic ulcer disease is not likely to be entirely genetic. The observed familial patterns appear to be due to shared infections with *H pylori*. Common gastrointestinal ailments are illustrated in ▲ **Figure 5-15.**

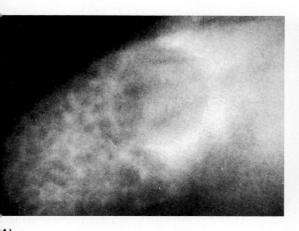

A)

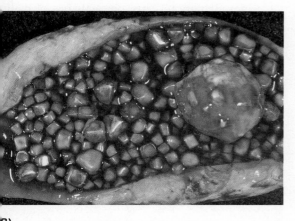

B)

Figure 5-16 **A.** Radiograph of gallbladder. Gallstones emonstrated by means of contrast material concentrated in ile. Gallstones occupy space and appear as dark areas within hite. Note large black area, indicating a large gallstone, urrounded by smaller black areas, representing multiple maller stones. **B.** Opened gallbladder removed surgically from e same patient.

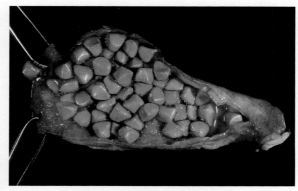

Figure 5-17 Opened gallbladder filled with gallstones composed of cholesterol.

Gallstones (cholethiasis) are stonelike masses in he gallbladder or its ducts caused by precipitation f substances contained in bile such as cholesterol nd bilirubin (▲ Figure 5-16). The following three fac- ors contribute to the formation of gallstones:

1. Abnormalities in the composition of bile
2. Stasis of bile
3. Inflammation of the gallbladder with many gallstones

allstones may be asymptomatic. Stones cause ymptoms when they obstruct the flow of bile. Small tones that are able to pass into the common duct roduce indigestion and biliary colic. Biliary colic ain is sudden in onset and increases steadily to its maximum in approximately an hour. The pain is located in the upper right quadrant or the epigastric area and may be referred to the back. Larger stones (▲ Figure 5-17) can obstruct the flow of bile and cause jaundice (yellow skin and sclerae). Genetic factors are responsible for at least 30% of symptomatic gall- stone disease. However, the true role of heredity in gallstone pathogenesis is probably higher because data based on symptomatic gallbladder disease underestimate the true prevalence in the population.

Obesity has become an epidemic in the United States. Obesity is an unhealthy accumulation of body fat. Its many deleterious side effects, both medical and social, are well-known. Health risks associated with obesity include hypertension, hyperlipidemia, cardiovascular disease, glucose intolerance, insulin resistance, diabetes, gallbladder disease, infertility, and cancer of the endometrium, breast, prostate, and colon. Current research sug- gests that a genetic predisposition is likely, but the role of specific genes has yet to be determined.

Neuromuscular Disorders

Although environmental contributions are highly likely, certain neuromuscular disorders have a famil- ial and genetic basis. Huntington's disease (also called Huntington's chorea) is an abnormal heredi- tary condition (autosomal dominant) characterized by progressive chorea (involuntary rapid, jerky motions) and mental deterioration, leading to dementia. Symptoms usually first appear in the third or fourth decade of life and progress to death, often within 15 years.

Muscular dystrophy is a generic term for any of a group of hereditary diseases of the muscular system characterized by weakness and wasting of groups of skeletal muscles, leading to increasing disability. The various forms differ in age of onset, rate of progression, and mode of genetic transmission. The most common is Duchenne's muscular dystrophy, a sex-linked recessive disease (affecting only males), with symptoms first appearing around the age of 4 years. Progressive wasting of leg and pelvic muscles produces a waddling gait and abnormal curvature of the spine, progressing to inability to walk and confinement to a wheelchair, usually by age 12 years. There is no specific treatment, and death, usually from heart disorders, often results by age 20 years.

Multiple sclerosis is progressive disease in which nerve fibers of the brain and spinal cord lose their myelin cover. It begins usually in early adulthood and progresses slowly, with periods of remission and exacerbation. Early symptoms of abnormal sensations in the face or extremities, weakness, and visual disturbances (eg, double vision) progress to ataxia (lack of coordination), abnormal reflexes, tremors, difficulty in urination, and difficulty in walking. Depression is also common. There is no specific treatment or cure; corticosteroids and other drugs are used to treat symptoms. Although multiple sclerosis is not directly inherited, there is a familial predisposition in some cases, suggesting a genetic influence on susceptibility.

Alzheimer's disease affects nearly four million Americans. Although the cause is unknown, the result is cortical atrophy and a loss of neurons in the frontal and temporal lobes of the brain. Atrophy occurs and there is ventricular enlargement due to the loss of brain tissue. The histologic changes in the brain of an Alzheimer's patient include neurofibrillary tangles and senile plaques (▼ Figure 5-18). Studies on the genetics of inherited early onset Alzheimer's have been linked to mutations on three genes. Clinical manifestations follow three distinct stages:

1. Stage 1 – memory loss, lack of spontaneity, subtle personality changes, and disorientation to time and date.
2. Stage 2 – impaired cognition and abstract thinking, restlessness and agitation, wandering, inability to carry out activities of daily living, impaired judgment, inappropriate social behavior.
3. Stage 3 – indifference to food, inability to communicate, urinary and fecal incontinence, seizures.

Psychiatric Disorders

Although all the details remain to be worked out, data support a familial, and perhaps even genetic, component to some common psychiatric disorders.

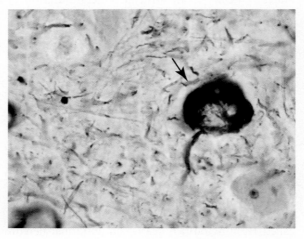

(A)

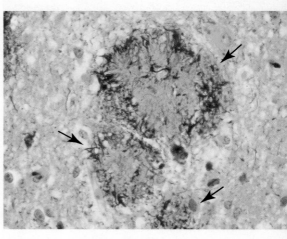

(B)

Figure 5-18 Alzheimer's disease. **A.** Thickened neurofilaments encircle and obscure nucleus of nerve cells (*arrow*) forming neurofibrillary tangle (silver stain; original magnification, ×400). **B.** Three senile plaques (*arrows*), composed of broken masses of thickened neurofilaments (silver stain; original magnification, ×100).

Special Needs

Never assume that new or worsening confusion in a geriatric patient is due purely to Alzheimer's disease. The paramedic should always consider potentially correctable causes such as new medications, infections, or myocardial infarction.

The paramedic should always consider that there may be an organic cause of an "apparent" emotional, psychological, or behavioral problem. This is especially true in the geriatric population. The most common cause of these incidents or outbreaks are medication (eg, drug-induced sedation or psychosis), severe infection, and hypoxia from any cause.

Case Study

Case Study, Part 4

Completion of Case Study

While en route to the hospital, you learned from the patient that the simplest treatment for hemochromatosis is phlebotomy. The regular blood drawing often helped his symptoms but obviously does not prevent the development of cancer. However, not every patient who has this disorder develops liver cancer.

CASE STUDY

Physiology

Diseases such as cystic fibrosis, muscular dystrophy, and Huntington's disease are single-gene disorders. If a person inherits a gene that causes one of these disorders, the disease will usually develop. Alzheimer's disease, on the other hand, is not caused by a single gene. More than one gene mutation can cause Alzheimer's disease, and genes on multiple chromosomes are involved.

The two basic types of Alzheimer's disease are familial and sporadic. Familial Alzheimer's disease (FAD) is a rare form of Alzheimer's disease, affecting less than 10% of patients with Alzheimer's disease. FAD is early onset, meaning the disease typically develops before age 65 years. It is caused by gene mutations on chromosomes 1, 14, and 21. If even one of these mutated genes is inherited from a parent, the person will almost always develop early onset Alzheimer's disease. This inheritance pattern is referred to as autosomal dominant inheritance. In other words, all offspring within the same generation have at least a 50% chance of developing FAD if one of their parents had the disease.

The majority of cases of Alzheimer's disease are sporadic, meaning they have no known cause. Because this type of Alzheimer's disease usually develops after age 65 years, it often is referred to as late-onset Alzheimer's disease. Sporadic Alzheimer's disease shows no obvious inheritance pattern; however, in some families, clusters of cases have been seen. Although a specific gene has not been identified as the cause of sporadic Alzheimer's disease, genetics does appear to play a role in the development of this form of the disease. Researchers have identified an increased risk of developing sporadic Alzheimer's disease associated with the apolipoprotein E (apoE) gene found on chromosome 19. This gene codes for a protein that helps carry cholesterol in the bloodstream. ApoE comes in several different forms, or genes, but three occur most frequently: apoE2 (E2), apoE3 (E3), and apoE4 (E4).

People inherit one apoE gene from each parent. Having one or two copies of the E4 gene increases a person's risk of Alzheimer's disease. That is, having the E4 gene is a risk factor for Alzheimer's disease, but not a certainty. Some people with two copies of the E4 gene (the highest risk group) do not develop the disease, while others without the E4 genes do. The rarer E2 gene appears to be associated with a lower risk of Alzheimer's disease. The E3 gene is the most common form found in the general population and may play a neutral role. The exact degree of risk of the disease for any given person cannot be determined based on apoE status.

<u>Schizophrenia</u> is any of a group of mental disorders characterized by gross distortions of reality (psychoses), withdrawal from social contacts, and disturbances of thought, language, perception, and emotional response. Symptoms are highly varied and may include apathy, catatonia, or excessive activity, bizarre actions, hallucinations, delusions, and rambling speech. There is no known cause; a combination of hereditary or genetic predisposing factors is likely in most cases.

<u>Manic-depressive disorder</u>, also known as bipolar disorder or manic-depressive psychosis, is a mental disorder characterized by episodes of mania and depression. One or the other phase may be dominant at a given time, and the phases may alternate or aspects of both phases may be present at the same time. Treatment is by psychotherapy and the use of antidepressants and tranquilizers. The higher rates of bipolar disorder among relatives, identical twins, and

Paramedic Safety Tip

Do not turn your back on patients who present with a behavioral emergency, especially those who have been diagnosed with a bipolar disorder. Be sensitive and compassionate and listen to their story and concerns, **but** remember that their affect can change quickly and radically, and in some cases they may become a threat to your personal safety.

biologic parents relative to adoptive parents have all been cited as evidence of the role of genetics in this disorder. These higher risks are measured relative to a roughly 1% risk of the disorder occurring within the general population as a whole.

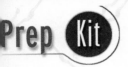

Chapter Summary

- Age and sex-associated factors interact with a combination of genetic and environmental factors, lifestyle, and anatomic or hormonal differences to cause disease. Some diseases are more prevalent in men, such as lung cancer, gout, and Parkinson's disease. Women are more likely to experience osteoporosis, rheumatoid arthritis, and breast cancer.

- Analyzing disease risk involves consideration of disease rates (incidence, prevalence, mortality) and disease risk factors (both causal and noncausal). There is typically much interaction between risk factors, age, and sex differences.

- A true genetic risk is one that is passed through generations on a gene. This is not always the case for a familial tendency, which may "cluster" in family groups despite lack of evidence for heritable gene-associated abnormalities. In autosomal dominant inheritance, a person only needs to inherit one copy of a particular form of a gene in order to show that trait. It does not matter what form of the gene that person inherits from the other parent. A parent has at least a 50% chance of passing on an autosomal dominant inherited condition to his or her child. In autosomal recessive inheritance, you must inherit two copies of a particular form of a gene in order to show that trait. A parent has up to a 50% chance of passing on an autosomal recessive inherited condition to his or her child if he or she exhibits the disease and the other parent does not.

- Immunologic diseases occur because of hyperactivity or hypoactivity of the immune system. Allergies are acquired following initial exposure to a stimulant, known as an allergen. Repeated exposures cause a reaction by the immune system to the allergen. Asthma is a chronic, inflammatory condition resulting in intermittent wheezing and excess mucus production. Rheumatic fever is an inflammatory disease, occurring primarily in children, resulting in delayed reaction to an inadequately treated streptococcal infection of the upper respiratory tract. A family history of acute rheumatic fever may predispose an individual to the disease.

- Cancer is a general term to describe a large number of malignant neoplasms. The prognosis depends on aggressiveness of the particular tumor, extent of its spread when found including presence or absence of metastases, and the effectiveness of treatment. Lung cancer is the leading cause of death from cancer, with its major risk factor being cigarette smoking. Other forms of cancer also have a familial tendency. Women whose first-degree relatives (ie, parent, sister, daughter) have breast cancer are 2.1 times as likely to develop the disease. Risk varies with the age at which the affected relative was diagnosed: the younger the affected relative, the greater the risk posed to relatives. Approximately 5% to 10% of patients with breast cancer demonstrate a pattern of autosomal dominant inheritance. Relatives of people who have had colorectal cancer are more likely to develop the disease themselves.

- There are two major forms of diabetes mellitus: ketoacidosis prone and nonketoacidosis prone. Both forms have a hereditary predisposition.

- Hematologic disorders that show a familial or genetic predisposition include hemolytic anemia, hemophilia, and hematochromatosis.

- Several cardiovascular disorders are known to follow specific patterns of inheritance (eg, autosomal dominant, autosomal recessive). Still others have strong familial tendencies (eg, coronary heart disease). These include long QT syndrome, cardiomyopathy, MVP, coronary heart disease, and stroke.

- Gout is an abnormal accumulation of uric acid due to a defect in its metabolism. As a result, uric acid accumulates in the blood and joints, causing pain and swelling of the joints, especially the big toe. Gout usually has a genetic basis. Kidney stones are small masses of uric acid or calcium salts that form in any part of the urinary system (eg, kidney, ureter, bladder) and often have a genetic basis.

- Malabsorption disorders result from defects in the function of the bowel wall preventing normal absorption of nutrients. Those with a familial or genetic component include lactose intolerance, ulcerative colitis, and Crohn's disease. Peptic ulcers are circumscribed erosions in the mucous membrane lining of the gastrointestinal tract. They may occur in the esophagus, stomach, duodenum, or jejunum. Peptic ulcer disease is not currently believed to be wholly genetic. The observed familial patterns are thought due to shared infections with *H pylori*.

- Gallstones (cholethiasis) are stonelike masses in the gallbladder or its ducts caused by precipitation of substances contained in bile such as cholesterol and bilirubin. Genetic factors are responsible for at least 30% of symptomatic gallstone disease.

- Obesity has become an epidemic in the United States. Current research indicates that a genetic component is likely, but the role of specific genes has not yet been determined.

- Although environmental contributions are highly likely, certain neuromuscular disorders have a familial and genetic basis, such as Huntington's disease, muscular dystrophy, multiple sclerosis, and Alzheimer's disease.

- Data support a familial, and perhaps even genetic, component to some common psychiatric disorders, such as schizophrenia and manic-depressive disorder.

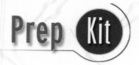

Vital Vocabulary

allergen A stimulant or agent that causes an allergy.

Alzheimer's disease A disease that results in cortical atrophy and loss of neurons in the frontal and temporal lobes of the brain.

asthma A chronic inflammatory lower airway condition resulting in intermittent wheezing and excess mucus production.

atopic The medical term for having an allergic tendency.

autosomal dominant A pattern of inheritance that involves genes that are located on autosomes or the nonsex chromosomes. You only need to inherit a single copy of a particular form of a gene in order to show the trait.

autosomal recessive A pattern of inheritance that involves genes located on autosomes or the nonsex chromosomes. You must inherit two copies of a particular form of a gene to show the trait.

cardiomyopathy A general term for disease of the myocardium that ultimately progresses to heart failure, acute myocardial infarction, or death. The heart muscle becomes thin, flabby, dilated, or enlarged.

coronary heart disease A disease caused by impaired circulation to the heart; also called coronary artery disease.

Crohn's disease A chronic inflammatory condition affecting the colon and terminal part of the small intestine.

diabetes mellitus A chronic disorder of metabolism due to either partial or total lack of insulin secretion by the pancreas.

gallstones Stonelike masses in the gallbladder or its ducts caused by precipitation of substances contained in bile such as cholesterol and bilirubin; also called cholethiasis.

gout An abnormal accumulation of uric acid due to a defect in its metabolism. This causes an accumulation of acid in the joints and blood, causing pain and swelling especially to the big toe.

Helicobacter pylori The bacterium thought to be a major contributor to the development of peptic ulcers.

hemochromatosis An inherited disease in which the body absorbs more iron than it needs and stores it in the liver, kidneys, and pancreas.

hemolytic anemia A disease characterized by increased destruction of the red blood cells. It can occur from an Rh factor reaction, exposure to chemicals, or a disorder of the immune system.

hemophilia An inherited sex-linked disorder characterized by excessive bleeding.

Huntington's disease An abnormal hereditary condition characterized by progressive involuntary rapid, jerky motions, and mental deterioration leading to dementia; also known as Huntington's chorea.

hypercholesterolemia An elevated blood cholesterol level.

hypertrophic cardiomyopathy An inherited cardiomyopathy that causes an excessive thickening of the heart muscle.

incidence The frequency with which a disease occurs.

kidney stones Small masses of uric acid or calcium salts that form in the urinary system when uric acid accumulates in the kidney.

lactose intolerance A defect or deficiency of the enzyme lactase resulting in an inability to digest lactose.

long QT syndrome An inherited cardiac conduction system abnormality resulting in a prolongation of the QT interval on the ECG.

malabsorption disorders Disorders caused by a defect in the function of the bowel wall that prevents normal absorption of nutrients.

manic-depressive disorder Also called bipolar disorder or manic-depressive psychosis, this mental disorder is characterized by episodes of mania and depression.

mitral valve prolapse (MVP) Often referred to as a floppy mitral valve, this condition is characterized by mitral valve leaflets that balloon into the left atrium during systole.

mortality The number of deaths from a disease in a given population.

multiple sclerosis A progressive disease in which nerve fibers of the brain and spinal cord lose their myelin cover. The disease begins in early adulthood and progresses slowly with periods of remission and exacerbation.

muscular dystrophy A generic term for any of a group of hereditary diseases of the muscular system characterized by weakness and wasting of groups of skeletal muscles.

obesity An unhealthy accumulation of body fat in which the body mass index is greater than 30 kg/m².

peptic ulcer disease A disease associated with erosions in the mucous membrane lining the gastrointestinal tract.

prevalence The number of cases in a specific population over time.

rheumatic fever An inflammatory disease that is a result of a delayed reaction to an untreated streptococcal infection of the upper respiratory tract.

schizophrenia A group of mental disorders characterized by gross distortions of reality, withdrawal from societal contacts, and disturbances of thought, language, perception, and emotional response.

type 1 diabetes The form of diabetes with which patients need exogenous insulin to live; also called ketoacidosis prone diabetes.

type 2 diabetes The form of diabetes that is often controlled by diet and/or oral antidiabetic medications; also called nonketoacidosis prone diabetes.

ulcerative colitis A serious chronic inflammatory disease of the large intestine and rectum.

Case Study Answers

Question 1: What are the causes of cancer?

Answer: Cancers are caused by more than one process. Genetics, biologic factors, environmental factors, age, and sex are all believed to play a role in the alteration of the cell's DNA that leads to cancer.

Question 2: Are all of the patient's medical problems related to cancer?

Answer: Hemochromatosis involves chronic iron overload, which causes the body to absorb more iron than it requires. It is an inherited disease. The total body iron content can reach as high as 50 g, compared with the normal levels of 3.5 g in males and 2.5 g in females. This disease can lead to other diseases including hepatitis C, liver disease and cancer, diabetes, and heart disease.

Question 3: How is hemochromatosis passed from one generation to the next?

Answer: Hemochromatosis is inherited from both parents carrying a mutated copy of the gene, or in an autosomal recessive manner.

Question 4: How is the prognosis for cancer determined?

Answer: The prognosis for cancer depends on the tissue involved, the extent of the growth when first discovered, and the effectiveness of the treatment and the aggressiveness of the particular tumor diagnosed. The prognosis for liver cancer is usually not good, and treatment is generally unsatisfactory.

Question 5: Is liver cancer one of the leading causes of death from cancer?

Answer: No, lung cancer is the leading cause of death from cancer. Breast cancer is the second leading cause of death in women, and colorectal cancer is the third most common cause of death in both males and females.

Question 6: What are some of the environmental factors that may have contributed to the development of this patient's cancer?

Answer: Environmental factors include microorganisms, immunologic and toxic exposures, personal habits and lifestyle, exposures to chemicals, physical environment, and the psychosocial environment. The exact cause of the conversion of normal cells into cancerous ones is still not fully understood.

Question 7: What is type 2 diabetes and is it hereditary?

Answer: Type 2 diabetes (nonketoacidosis prone) is considered non-insulin-dependent diabetes, although many type 2 diabetics still require exogenous insulin injections to survive. Both type 1 and type 2 diabetes have a hereditary predisposition.

CASE STUDY ANSWERS

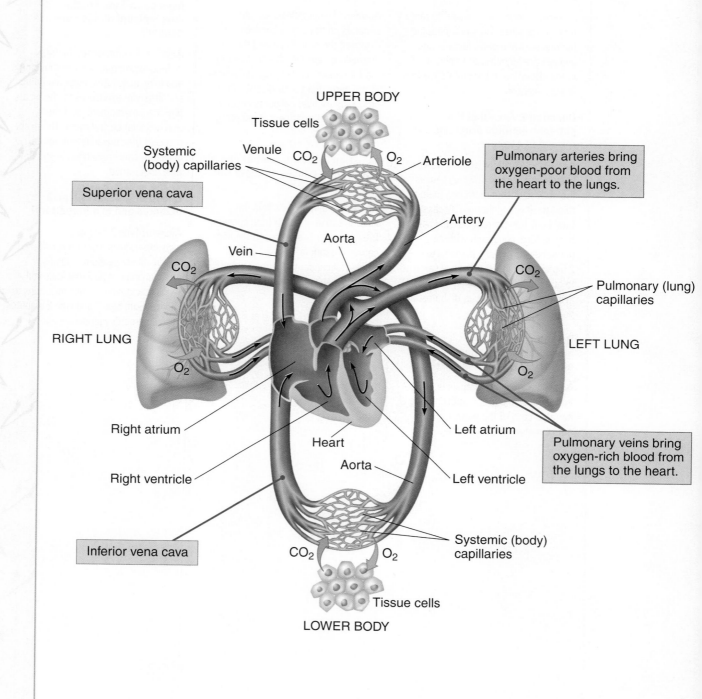

UPPER BODY

Tissue cells

Systemic (body) capillaries

Venule

CO_2

O_2

Arteriole

Superior vena cava

Vein

Aorta

Artery

Pulmonary arteries bring oxygen-poor blood from the heart to the lungs.

CO_2

CO_2

RIGHT LUNG

O_2

O_2

LEFT LUNG

Pulmonary (lung) capillaries

Right atrium

Heart

Left atrium

Right ventricle

Aorta

Left ventricle

Pulmonary veins bring oxygen-rich blood from the lungs to the heart.

Inferior vena cava

CO_2

O_2

Systemic (body) capillaries

Tissue cells

LOWER BODY

Hypoperfusion

6

OBJECTIVES

Cognitive

1-6.10 Discuss hypoperfusion. (p 96)

1-6.11 Define cardiogenic, hypovolemic, neurogenic, anaphylactic and septic shock. (p 98–100)

1-6.12 Describe multiple organ dysfunction syndrome. (p 102)

TECHNOLOGY

www.Paramedic.EMSzone.com

- Online Chapter Pretest
- Vocabulary Explorer
- Anatomy Review
- Web Links

Chapter FEATURES

- Case Studies
- Physiology Tips
- Medication Tips
- Paramedic Safety Tips
- Special Needs Tips
- Vital Vocabulary
- Prep Kit

Pathogenesis

<u>Perfusion</u> is defined as delivery of oxygen and nutrients, and removal of wastes, from the cells, organs, and tissues by the circulatory system. Evaluation of a patient's level of organ perfusion is important in emergency care, especially in diagnosing shock. <u>Hypoperfusion</u> occurs when the level of tissue perfusion decreases below normal.

When the body senses tissue hypoperfusion, compensatory mechanisms are set into motion. In some cases, this is all that is required to stabilize the patient. Often, however, the severity of disease or injury overwhelms the normal compensatory mechanisms and the patient's condition progressively deteriorates.

In response to hypoperfusion, catecholamines (ie, epinephrine and norepinephrine) are released. These cause vasoconstriction (increased systemic vascular resistance). In addition, the renin-angiotensin-aldosterone system is activated and antidiuretic hormone is released from the pituitary gland. Together these trigger salt and water retention as well as peripheral vasoconstriction. The result is an increase in blood pressure and cardiac output. Depending on the severity of the insult, variable amounts of fluid will shift from the interstitial tissues into the vascular compartment. The spleen also releases some red blood cells that are normally sequestered ("kept") there to augment the oxygen-carrying capacity of the blood. The overall response of the initial compensatory mechanisms is to increase the preload (venous return), stroke volume, and heart rate. The result is usually an increase in cardiac output and an increase in myocardial oxygen demand. The signs and symptoms found in the compensated and decompensated phases of hypoperfusion are listed in ▼ **Table 6-1**.

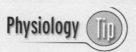

Physiology Tip

Early decreased tissue perfusion may result in subtle changes, such as agitation or restlessness, prior to development of abnormality in a patient's vital signs (eg, decreased blood pressure and elevated pulse or respiratory rate).

As hypoperfusion persists, the myocardial oxygen demand continues to increase. Eventually, the above-normal compensatory mechanisms are no longer able to keep up with the demand. As a result, myocardial function worsens, with decreased cardiac output and ejection fraction. Tissue perfusion decreases, leading to impaired cell metabolism. Often, the blood pressure decreases, especially in progressive hypoperfusion. Fluid may leak from the blood vessels, causing systemic and pulmonary edema. At this point, other signs of hypoperfusion may be present, such as dusky skin, oliguria, and impaired mentation.

Types of Shock

<u>Shock</u> is an abnormal state associated with inadequate oxygen and nutrient delivery to the metabolic apparatus of the cell. The result is an impairment of cell metabolism. Once a certain level of tissue hypoperfusion is reached, cell damage proceeds in a similar manner regardless of the type of initial insult. Impairment of cellular metabolism results in the inability to properly use oxygen and glucose at the cellular level. The cell converts to anaerobic

Table 6-1

Signs and Symptoms in the Compensated and Decompensated Phases of Hypoperfusion

Compensated Hypoperfusion	Decompensated Hypoperfusion
Agitation, anxiety, restlessness	Altered mental status (verbal to unresponsive)
Sense of impending doom	Hypotension
Weak, rapid (thready) pulse	Labored or irregular breathing
Clammy (cool, moist) skin	Thready or absent peripheral pulses
Pallor with cyanotic lips	Ashen, mottled, or cyanotic skin
Shortness of breath	Dilated pupils
Nausea, vomiting	Diminished urine output (oliguria)
Delayed capillary refill in infants and children	Impending cardiac arrest
Thirst	
Normal systolic blood pressure	

Physiology Tip

The terms shock and hypoperfusion are usually synonymous, at least when they are applied to multiple body systems. Localized hypoperfusion, such as from arterial occlusion, is *not* shock.

Medication Tip

The body produces its own "medicines," which are released by the adrenal glands in response to hypoperfusion—epinephrine and norepinephrine. They are released by the body as part of the global compensatory state, but they fail to work as hypoperfusion persists. Release of epinephrine improves cardiac output by increasing the heart rate and strength. Norepinephrine triggers vasoconstriction, which allows the body to shunt blood from areas of lesser need to areas of greater need. In an effort to maintain circulation to the brain, the body will shunt blood away from other less critical organs, including the placenta, skin, muscles, gut, kidneys, liver, heart, and lungs. The skin and muscles can survive with minimal blood flow from vasoconstriction for a much longer period of time than major organs such as the kidneys, liver, heart, and lungs. If the blood supply is inadequate to the major organs for more than 60 minutes, they often develop complications that can lead to overall deterioration, such as renal failure and acute lung injury. This is why it is so important to address the underlying cause of the shock as quickly as possible. Aside from the release of the body's own epinephrine and norepinephrine, epinephrine is administered in cases of anaphylaxis, severe airway disease, and cardiac arrest. ▼ Figure 6-1 shows an epinephrine auto-injector, which is used in the out-of-hospital setting. Norepinephrine is not commonly administered in hypoperfusion, except in cases of septic shock.

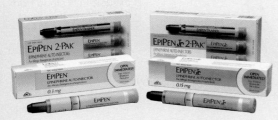

Figure 6-1 Patients who are allergic to bee stings often carry commercial bee sting kits, such as an IM injector or auto-injector, containing epinephrine.

Case Study

Case Study, Part 1

Your unit is dispatched to a motor vehicle collision at an intersection on a high-speed road. Three weeks ago a traffic light was installed at this intersection and since then several collisions have occurred there. Your call is for a patient with chest pain and difficulty breathing. When you arrive at the scene, you note that the first due engine company has identified two vehicles with significant front-end damage and started extrication of one trapped individual. A fire fighter is immobilizing the patient, who is wearing an oxygen mask.

Your general impression is that the patient is an older male, approximately 75 years old, who is disoriented, pale, having difficulty breathing, and complaining of chest pain. He is a high-priority patient who is going to need a rapid extrication and transport to the nearest trauma hospital.

Initial Assessment

Recording time
0 minutes

Appearance
Disoriented

Level of consciousness
Verbal—conscious but confused

Airway
Open

Vital Signs

Pulse rate/quality
100 beats/min, regular, strong

Blood pressure
110/50 mm Hg

Respiratory rate/depth
24 breaths/min, labored

Question 1: Is the patient showing any signs of shock? If so, what are they?

Question 2: What type of shock do you suspect the patient is experiencing?

Question 3: What happens when the body senses tissue hypoperfusion?

CASE STUDY

metabolism, which causes increased lactic acid production and metabolic acidosis, decreased oxygen affinity for hemoglobin, decreased adenosine triphosphate production, changes in cellular electrolytes, cellular edema, and release of lysosomal enzymes. Glucose impairment leads to elevated blood glucose levels due to release of catecholamines and cortisol. In addition, fat breakdown (lipolysis) with ketone formation may occur.

Shock can occur due to inadequacy of the central circulation (eg, the heart and the great vessels) or of the peripheral circulation (the remaining vessels, including the microscopic circulation [eg, arterioles, venules, and capillaries as illustrated in ▼ **Figure 6-2**]). From a mechanistic approach, there are two types of shock: central and peripheral. <u>Central shock</u> consists of cardiogenic shock and obstructive shock, while <u>peripheral shock</u> includes hypovolemic shock and distributive shock.

<u>Cardiogenic shock</u> occurs when the heart is unable to circulate sufficient blood to maintain adequate peripheral oxygen delivery. In the case of ischemic heart disease, this requires loss of 40% or more functioning myocardium. The most common cause of cardiogenic shock is myocardial infarction, either as a single event or by cumulative damage. Other forms of cardiac dysfunction may potentially result in cardiogenic shock (ie, large ventricular sep-

tal defect or hemodynamic significant dysrhythmias) (▶ **Figure 6-3**).

<u>Obstructive shock</u> occurs when there is a block to blood flow in the heart or great vessels. In pericardial tamponade (▶ **Figure 6-4**) diastolic filling of the right ventricle is impaired, leading to a decrease in the cardiac output. Aortic dissection leads to a false lumen (aortic opening) with loss of normal blood flow (▶ **Figure 6-5**). A left atrial tumor may obstruct flow between the atrium and ventricle and decrease cardiac output. Obstruction of either the superior or inferior vena cava (vena cava syndrome) decreases cardiac output by decreasing venous return. A large pulmonary embolus, or a tension pneumothorax, prevents adequate blood flow to the lungs, resulting in inadequate venous return to the left side of the heart.

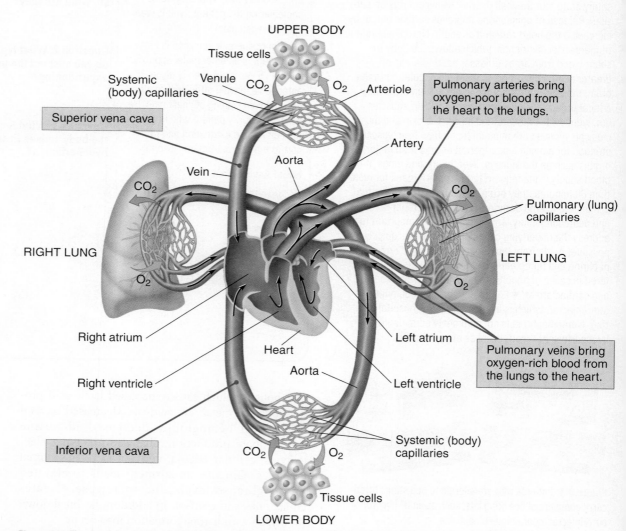

Figure 6-2 The circulatory system includes the heart, arteries, veins, and interconnecting capillaries. The capillaries are the smallest vessels and connect with the venules and arterioles. At the center of the system, and providing its driving force, is the heart.

Physiology (Tip)

In anaphylaxis, interstitial fluid may cause significant swelling. In some cases, this swelling may occlude the upper airway, resulting in a life-threatening condition. Recurrent large areas of subcutaneous edema of sudden onset, usually disappearing within 24 hours, is called angioedema. It is seen mainly in young women, frequently as a result of allergy to food or drugs.

<u>Hypovolemic shock</u> occurs when the circulating blood volume is unable to deliver adequate oxygen and nutrients to the body. There are two types of hypovolemic shock, exogenous and endogenous, depending on where the fluid loss occurs. The most common type of <u>exogenous hypovolemic shock</u> is external bleeding, such as from an open wound. Another example is loss of plasma volume caused by diarrhea or vomiting. <u>Endogenous hypovolemic shock</u> occurs when the fluid loss is contained within the body. In anaphylactic shock, histamine and other vasodilator proteins are released upon exposure to an allergen. Anaphylaxis is also accompanied by wheezing and <u>urticaria</u> (hives) (▶ **Figure 6-6**). The result is widespread vasodilation that causes distributive shock, as described below, and blood vessels that continue to leak. Fluid leaks out of the blood vessels into the interstitial spaces, resulting in intravascular hypovolemia.

<u>Distributive shock</u> occurs when there is widespread dilation of the <u>resistance vessels</u> (small arterioles), the <u>capacitance vessels</u> (small venules), or both. As a result, the circulating blood volume "pools" in the expanded vascular beds and tissue perfusion decreases. The three most common types of distributive shock are anaphylactic shock, septic shock, and neurogenic shock (▶ **Figure 6-7**).

Septic shock occurs as a result of widespread infection, usually bacterial. Complex interactions occur between the bacterial invader and the body's defense systems. Initially, our own defense mechanisms may keep the infection at bay. If the normal immune mechanisms are overwhelmed, a multitude of substances are produced, which cause vasodilation and decreased cardiac output. Untreated, the result is multiple organ dysfunction syndrome and often death.

Neurogenic shock usually results from spinal cord injury. The effect is loss of normal sympathetic nervous system tone and vasodilation. Often

Case Study

Case Study, Part 2

A cervical collar is placed on the patient, and he is rapidly extricated from the vehicle and moved to the ambulance. You ask the incident commander to assign an extra driver to your vehicle to allow both you and your partner to attend to this patient. Transport is started. It will be approximately 15 minutes to the trauma center. Inside the ambulance you remove the patient's clothing and perform a rapid assessment and a focused physical exam, treating life-threatening conditions as they are discovered. The patient's breathing is labored and breath sounds are decreased, especially on the right side. His distal pulse is becoming weak and remains fast. His skin is pale and moist. There are no apparent injuries to his head. His chest is tender on the right and the ribs are unstable. His abdomen is tender in the lower quadrants, and his pelvis is unstable. The extremities appear uninjured.

The patient is still confused about what has happened. You tell him what happened and what you are doing as you start two large-bore IVs. Your partner attaches the monitor and notifies the trauma center about the patient and the estimated time of arrival.

Focused Physical Assessment

Recording time
5 minutes

Mental status
Confused

Airway
Open

Breathing
Labored with decreased breath sounds

Circulation
Pale and moist skin, rapid, and weak pulse

Injuries
Chest injury, abdominal injury, and unstable pelvis

Vital Signs

Pulse rate/quality
110 beats/min, regular, weak

Blood pressure
100/48 mm Hg

Respiratory rate/depth
30 breaths/min, shallow and labored

Diagnostic Tools

Electrocardiogram
Sinus tachycardia

SpO2
93%

Blood glucose level
140 mg/dL

Question 4: What happens when hypoperfusion persists?

Question 5: What are the treatment goals in this type of injury?

CASE STUDY

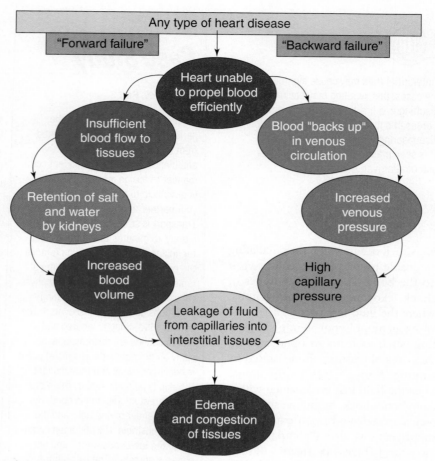

Figure 6-3 Mechanisms in the pathogenesis of congestive heart failure.

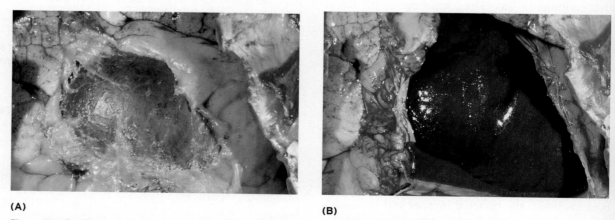

(A)   **(B)**

Figure 6-4 Cardiac tamponade secondary to myocardial rupture. **A.** Distended pericardial sac. **B.** Pericardial sac opened, showing clotted blood surrounding the heart, which compressed the heart and prevented filling of the right ventricle in diastole.

patients have fluid-refractory hypotension due to the degree of vasodilation.

Regardless of the type of shock, it is characterized by reduced cardiac output, circulatory insufficiency, and rapid heartbeat. Most types of shock also include pallor, except for spinal shock or sepsis. The patient's mental status may be altered. Although low blood pressure is classically associated with shock, it is a late sign, especially in children. Treatment primarily addresses the underlying condition. IV fluid therapy can be helpful in supplementing the initial therapies.

Physiology Tip

A possible exception to the rule of IV fluid therapy is hypovolemic shock caused by ongoing bleeding. Some studies are suggesting that fluid therapy to maintain the systolic blood pressure at approximately 80 mm Hg may be safer for the patient than to attempt restoration of normotension, which may aggravate ongoing bleeding. As always, follow your local protocols.

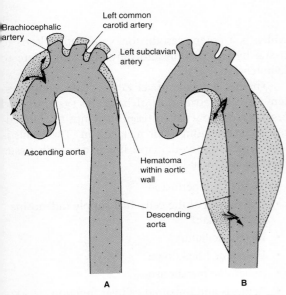

Figure 6-5 Sites of thoracic aortic dissection. **A.** A tear in the ascending aorta causes both proximal and distal dissection. **B.** A tear in the descending aorta may cause extensive distal dissection.

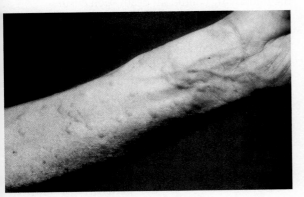

Figure 6-6 Urticaria, or hives, may appear following a sting and is characterized by multiple small, raised areas on the skin. Urticaria may be one of the warning signs of impending anaphylaxsis.

Case Study

Case Study, Part 3

Five minutes out from the trauma center the patient loses consciousness. As you prepare to intubate him, your partner reassesses his vital signs and injuries and gives the hospital an update.

Ongoing Assessment

Recording time
15 minutes

Mental status
Unresponsive

Airway/breathing
Intubated

Circulation
Pale, weak, and rapid pulse

Vital Signs

Pulse rate/quality
110 beats/min, regular, weak

Blood pressure
80/40 mm Hg after an infusion of 1.5 L of normal saline

Respiratory rate/depth
Good breath sounds with bagging

Diagnostic Tools

Electrocardiogram
Sinus tachycardia

SpO$_2$
95%

Question 6: What is multiple organ dysfunction syndrome? Is the patient experiencing this condition?

Question 7: Was the patient's age a contributing factor to his rapid deterioration?

CASE STUDY

Case Study

Case Study, Part 4

Completion of Case Study

Before the patient reaches the operating suite he goes into cardiac arrest. The emergency department staff worked aggressively on the patient for 20 minutes. Unfortunately, they were unsuccessful in restoring his pulse. Later you learned that the patient had sustained injury to his right lung, had fractured ribs, a lacerated liver, and a pelvic fracture. As you suspected, the patient had significant blood loss due to multiple system trauma. Older persons are at a great disadvantage when faced with a traumatic injury. As the body ages, body systems begin to deteriorate, resulting in serious impairment of physiologic reserve; this impairment can result in loss of ability to adequately compensate for both moderate and severe illness or injury.

CASE STUDY

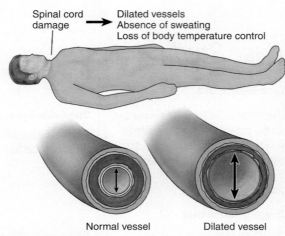

Spinal cord damage → Dilated vessels
Absence of sweating
Loss of body temperature control

Normal vessel   Dilated vessel

Figure 6-7 Damage to the spinal cord can cause significant injury to the part of the nervous system that controls the size and muscle tone of blood vessels. If the muscles in the blood vessels are cut off from their impulses to contract, then the vessels dilate widely, increasing the size and capacity of the vascular system. The blood in the body can no longer fill the enlarged vessels, resulting in inadequate perfusion in the form of neurogenic shock.

Multiple Organ Dysfunction Syndrome

<u>Multiple organ dysfunction syndrome (MODS)</u> is a progressive condition usually characterized by combined failure of several organs, such as the lungs, liver, and kidney, along with some clotting mechanisms, which occurs after severe illness or injury. First described in 1975, MODS has been associated with a mortality rate of 60% to 90%. It is the major cause of death following sepsis, trauma, and burn injuries. MODS is classified as either primary MODS or secondary MODS. <u>Primary MODS</u> is a direct result of an insult, such as a pulmonary contusion from striking the chest on the steering wheel during a collision. <u>Secondary MODS</u> is defined as the organ dysfunction that occurs as an integral component to the patient's response (eg, renal failure following trauma).

MODS occurs when injury or infection (eg, septic shock) triggers a massive systemic immune, inflammatory, and coagulation response with release of numerous inflammatory mediators. There is overactivation of the body's complement system causing increased inflammation and damage to the cells. MODS causes an overactivation of the body's coagulation system, due to endothelial damage, which in turn causes uncontrolled coagulation in the microscopic venules and arterioles. This results in microvascular thrombus formation and tissue ischemia.

MODS also causes activation of the kallikrein/kinin system, resulting in the release of bradykinin

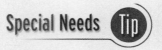

Special Needs Tip

In children, the immune system is not fully developed; on the other hand, the geriatric patient experiences decreased immune function as part of the normal aging process. As a result, both patient groups have an increased susceptibility to infection. This in turn is a common cause of MODS. The organs of the very old or very young patient have a limited physiologic reserve. Thus when organs begin to fail, serious problems are evident fairly early in the process.

which is a potent vasodilator. Vasodilation leads to tissue hypoperfusion and may also contribute to hypotension.

The net outcome of activation of the above systems is maldistribution of both the systemic and organ blood flow. Often tissues attempt to compensate by accelerating their metabolism. The result is an oxygen supply–demand imbalance with tissue hypoxia and includes:

- Tissue hypoperfusion
- Exhaustion of the cells' fuel supply (adenosine triphosphate)
- Metabolic failure
- Lysosome breakdown
- Anaerobic metabolism
- Acidosis and impaired cellular function

Cell and tissue hypoxia leads to organ dysfunction. As MODS progresses, various organs develop dysfunction. Renal failure and myocardial depression set in. If the patient does not respond to treatment of the underlying condition, death soon ensues.

MODS typically develops hours to days following resuscitation. The signs and symptoms of MODS include hypotension, insufficient tissue perfusion, uncontrollable bleeding (coagulopathy), and multisystem organ failure caused mainly by hypoxia, tissue acidosis, and severe local alterations of metabolism. Patients can have a low-grade fever from the inflammatory response, tachycardia, and dyspnea. Patients with MODS may be difficult to oxygenate due to the presence of acute lung injury and possibly adult respiratory distress syndrome.

During a 14- to 21-day period, renal and liver failure can develop in patients with MODS, along with collapse of the gastrointestinal and immune systems. Cardiovascular collapse and death typically occur within days to weeks of the initial insult.

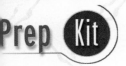

Chapter Summary

- Perfusion is defined as the delivery of oxygen and nutrients to cells, organs, and tissues through the circulatory system.

- Hypoperfusion occurs when the level of tissue perfusion decreases below normal. When the body senses tissue hypoperfusion, compensatory mechanisms are set into action. Often, however, the severity of disease or injury overwhelms the normal compensatory mechanisms and the patient's condition deteriorates.

- In response to hypoperfusion, catecholamines (ie, epinephrine and norepinephrine) are released into the circulation. These cause vasoconstriction (increased system vascular resistance). In addition, activation of the peripheral renin-angiotensin-aldosterone system and antidiuretic hormone released from the pituitary gland together trigger salt and water retention as well as increased peripheral vasoconstriction. The result is an increase in blood pressure and cardiac output. The overall response of the initial compensatory mechanisms is to increase the preload (venous return), stroke volume, and heart rate. The result is usually an increase in cardiac output. When normal compensatory mechanisms are insufficient, myocardial function worsens, with decreased cardiac output and ejection fraction.

- Shock is an abnormal state associated with inadequate oxygen and nutrient delivery to the metabolic apparatus of the cell. The result is an impairment of cell metabolism.

- Shock can occur due to inadequacy of the central circulation (eg, the heart and the great vessels) or of the peripheral circulation (the remaining vessels). There are two types of central shock (cardiogenic and obstructive) and two types of peripheral shock (hypovolemic and distributive).

- Cardiogenic shock occurs when the heart is unable to pump a sufficient amount of blood to maintain adequate oxygen delivery. Obstructive shock occurs when there is a block to blood flow in the heart or great vessels. Hypovolemic shock occurs when the circulating blood volume is inadequate to deliver adequate oxygen and nutrients to the body. Distributive shock occurs when there is widespread dilation of the resistance vessels (small arterioles), the capacitance vessels (small venules), or both.

- Regardless of the type of shock, it is characterized by reduced cardiac output, circulatory insufficiency, rapid heartbeat, and pallor. Treatment primarily addresses the underlying condition.

- Multiple organ dysfunction syndrome (MODS) is a progressive condition usually characterized by combined failure of several organs, such as the lungs, liver, and kidney, along with some clotting mechanisms, which occurs after severe illness or injury. MODS occurs when injury or infection (eg, septic shock) triggers a massive systemic immune, inflammatory, and coagulation response. Numerous inflammatory mediators are released due to activation of the complement, coagulation, and kallikrein/kinin systems. As MODS progresses, various organ systems become progressively dysfunctional. Renal failure and myocardial depression set in. Failure to correct the underlying condition almost universally results in the death of the patient.

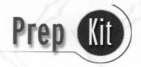

Vital Vocabulary

angioedema Recurrent large areas of subcutaneous edema of sudden onset, usually disappearing within 24 hours. Angioedema is seen mainly in young women, frequently as a result of allergy to food or drugs.

capacitance vessels Small venules.

cardiogenic shock A condition caused by loss of 40% or more of the functioning myocardium; the heart is no longer able to circulate sufficient blood to maintain adequate oxygen delivery.

central shock A term that describes shock secondary to central pump failure — includes both cardiogenic shock and obstructive shock.

distributive shock A condition that occurs when there is widespread dilation of the resistance vessels, the capacitance vessels, or both.

endogenous hypovolemic shock A condition that occurs when the fluid loss is contained within the body, such as in anaphylactic shock.

exogenous hypovolemic shock A condition that occurs when the fluid or blood loss is external or leaving the body.

hypoperfusion A condition that occurs when the level of tissue perfusion decreases below that needed to maintain normal cellular functions.

hypovolemic shock A condition that occurs when the circulating blood volume is inadequate to deliver adequate oxygen and nutrients to the body.

multiple organ dysfunction syndrome (MODS) A progressive condition usually characterized by combined failure of several organs, such as the lungs, liver, and kidney, along with some clotting mechanisms, which occurs after severe illness or injury.

obstructive shock A condition that occurs when there is a block to blood flow in the heart or great vessels causing an insufficient blood supply to the body's tissues.

perfusion The delivery of oxygen and nutrients to the cells, organs, and tissues of the body.

peripheral shock A term that describes shock secondary to peripheral circulatory abnormalities — includes both hypovolemic shock and distributive shock.

primary MODS The occurrence of MODS as a result of an insult, such as a pulmonary contusion from striking the chest on the steering wheel.

resistance vessels Small arterioles where constriction occurs to control peripheral vascular resistance.

secondary MODS Organ dysfunction that occurs as an integral component of the host's response.

shock An abnormal state associated with inadequate oxygen and nutrient delivery to the metabolic apparatus of the cell.

urticaria Multiple small, raised areas on the skin that may be one of the warning signs of impending anaphylaxsis. Also known as hives.

Case Study Answers

Question 1: Is the patient showing any signs of shock? If so, what are they?

Answer: The patient is showing early signs of shock. He is confused, which could be either a sign of cerebral hypoxia or of traumatic brain injury. His skin is pale, and his vital signs are showing signs of compensated shock with an increased pulse rate. The difficulty breathing and chest pain could be a chest injury and/or myocardial demand for more oxygen. A falling blood pressure is a late sign of shock. Because the patient's normal blood pressure is not known, it is unclear if he is hypotensive at this point.

Question 2: What type of shock do you suspect the patient is experiencing?

Answer: With the mechanism of injury being a high-speed collision with significant vehicle damage, you should suspect that the patient is in hypovolemic shock. We do not know yet what caused the collision. The patient may have had chest pain prior to the collision, making it a contributing factor. It is possible that he is in both cardiogenic shock and hypovolemic shock.

Question 3: What happens when the body senses tissue hypoperfusion?

Answer: When the body senses tissue hypoperfusion, compensatory mechanisms begin to kick in. The brain receives a message from the baroreceptors, located within the aortic arch and carotid sinus, that there is a subtle change in the pressure. This causes the brain to send a message along the spinal cord to the adrenal gland (located on top of the kidneys), stimulating the release of the catecholamines (ie, epinephrine and norepinephrine). These substances cause vasoconstriction of the blood vessels in the periphery. The impact on the heart is an increase in the rate and strength of contraction, which helps increase the cardiac output. Renin-angiotensin-aldosterone and antidiuretic hormones are also released, resulting in salt and water retention and additional vasoconstriction. These mechanisms are a physiologic attempt to maintain the blood pressure and brain perfusion by augmenting cardiac output.

Question 4: What happens when hypoperfusion persists?

Answer: When hypoperfusion persists due to blood loss or any other type of shock, the normal compensatory mechanisms become overwhelmed and begin to fail. The myocardial oxygen demand will continue to increase and cardiac output will decrease. This will result in a decreased mental status, a drop in blood pressure, poor skin color, decreased urine output, and impaired cell metabolism.

Question 5: What are the treatment goals in this type of injury?

Answer: The patient needs the operating suite immediately to stop internal bleeding and receive a blood transfusion. Your goal as a paramedic is to recognize this need and get the patient to the trauma center as quickly as possible, providing high-flow oxygen and IV fluids en route.

Question 6: What is multiple organ dysfunction syndrome? Is the patient experiencing this condition?

Answer: Multiple organ dysfunction syndrome (MODS) is a condition associated with a high mortality rate following a severe injury or illness such as sepsis, trauma, or burn injuries. The condition is progressive and is characterized by combined failure of several organs.

Question 7: Was the patient's age a contributing factor to his rapid deterioration?

Answer: There are special considerations for assessing the elderly trauma patient. Preexisting medical conditions may precipitate a traumatic injury, while chronic and degenerative disease processes can make an injury, even a minor one, worse. Cardiac stroke volume, respiratory capacities, and immune and thermoregulatory systems all deteriorate with age, thus giving the elderly patient a great disadvantage to compensate for a moderate to severe traumatic injury or illness.

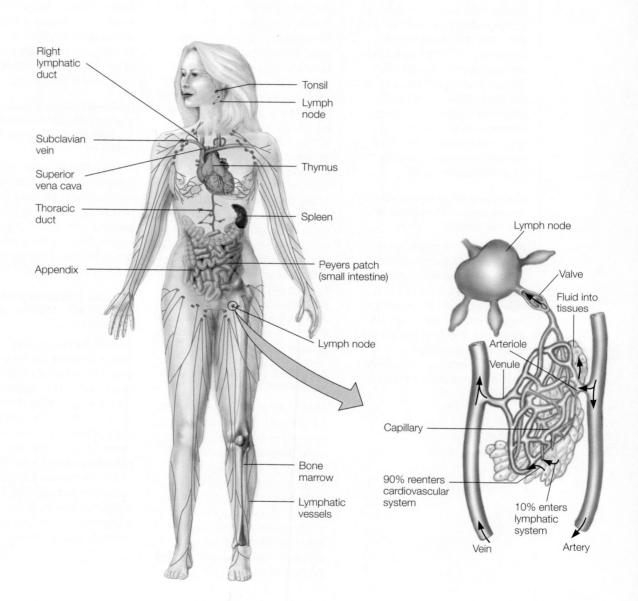

Right lymphatic duct

Tonsil

Lymph node

Subclavian vein

Superior vena cava

Thymus

Thoracic duct

Spleen

Appendix

Peyers patch (small intestine)

Lymph node

Bone marrow

Lymphatic vessels

Lymph node

Valve

Fluid into tissues

Arteriole

Venule

Capillary

90% reenters cardiovascular system

10% enters lymphatic system

Vein

Artery

Self-Defense Mechanisms

7

OBJECTIVES

Cognitive

-6.13 Define the characteristics of the immune response. (p 108)

-6.14 Discuss induction of the immune system. (p 113)

-6.15 Discuss fetal and neonatal immune function. (p 120)

-6.16 Discuss aging and the immune function in the elderly. (p 121)

Additional Objectives*

1. Summarize the humoral immune response. (p 115)

2. Summarize the cell-mediated immune response. (p 119)

3. Discuss interactions between innate and acquired immunity in bacterial infection. (p 120)

*These are noncurriculum objectives.

---

www.Paramedic.EMSzone.com

TECHNOLOGY

- Online Chapter Pretest
- Vocabulary Explorer
- Anatomy Review
- Web Links

Chapter FEATURES

- Case Studies
- Physiology Tips
- Medication Tips
- Paramedic Safety Tips
- Special Needs Tips
- Vital Vocabulary
- Prep Kit

Introduction: The Lines of Defense

The <u>immune system</u> includes all of the structures and processes associated with the body's defense against foreign substances and disease-causing agents. The body has three lines of defense:

1. Anatomic barriers – Several anatomic barriers decrease the chances of bodily invasion by foreign substances. The skin serves as a major deterrent. In addition, large and small hairs in the upper respiratory tract (the nose) and the lining of the lower respiratory tract (cilia-covered epithelial cells) help repel foreign matter, especially small particles and some bacteria. Acid in the stomach prevents many forms of infection from entering the body via the gastrointestinal tract.

2. Inflammatory response – The inflammatory response is a response of the tissues of the body to irritation or injury characterized by pain, swelling, redness, and heat. White blood cells of various types are a major component of this response (see Chapter 8, Inflammation). The inflammatory reaction and the immune response are independent processes, although they often occur simultaneously. Inflammation, however, can be present without activation of the immune response, and vice versa.

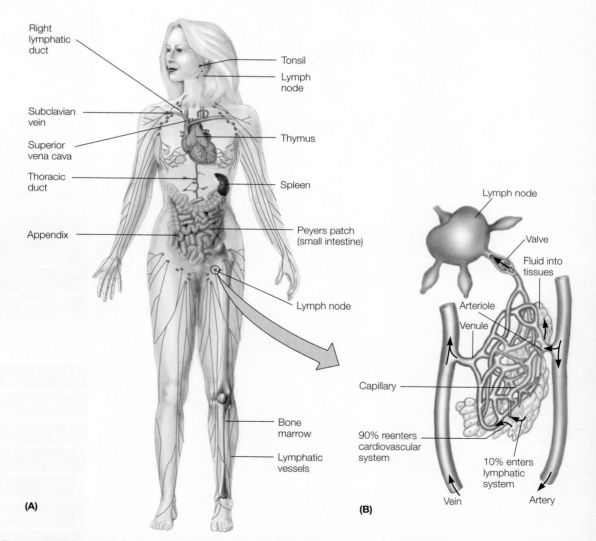

Figure 7-1 The lymphatic system. **A.** The lymphatic system consists of vessels that transport lymph and excess tissue fluid back to the circulatory system. **B.** Lymph is picked up by lymphatic capillaries that drain into larger vessels. Like the veins, the lymphatic vessels contain valves that prohibit backflow. Lymph nodes are interspersed along the vessels and serve to filter the lymph.

Physiology (Tip)

B lymphocytes originate from the same stem cells that give rise to all blood cell types. They mature in the bone marrow. T lymphocytes originate from the same bone marrow stem cells but travel to and mature in the thymus early in fetal life.

3. Immune response – The <u>immune response</u> is the body's defense reaction to any substance that is recognized as foreign. Often, this response is directed toward invading microbes, such as bacteria or viruses. However, the immune response is also triggered by foreign bodies (eg, a splinter) and even abnormal growths in our own cells (eg, a tumor).

Together, these three components of the immune system defend against foreign substances and disease-causing agents. Not all invaders can be destroyed by the body's immune system, however. In some cases, the best compromise the body can reach is to control the damage and keep the invader from spreading. Often, the immune system prevents severe disease following infection. When the normal systems become overwhelmed or fail, serious disease occurs.

Anatomy of the Immune System

The <u>lymphatic system</u> is a network of capillaries, vessels, ducts, nodes, and organs that help to maintain the fluid environment of the body by producing lymph and conveying it through the body (◄ Figure 7-1). The immune system has two anatomical components: the lymphoid tissues of the body and the cells that are responsible for the immune response.

Lymphoid tissues are distributed throughout the body. The two primary lymphoid tissues are the thymus gland and the bone marrow. Here cells involved in the immune response form and mature (► Figure 7-2). The <u>thymus gland</u> is a bilobed gland located below the thyroid gland and behind the sternum. It is prominent at birth and increases in size until the body reaches puberty. Then it becomes smaller and decreases in functional activity during adulthood. T lymphocytes originate from precursor cells in the bone marrow, leave the bone marrow, and mature in the thymus. The <u>bone marrow</u> is specialized soft tissue found within bone. Red bone marrow, widespread in the bones of children and found in some adult bones (eg, sternum, ribs), is

Case Study

Case Study, Part 1

Your unit is dispatched to a call for a severe allergic reaction from a bee sting. The dispatcher states that the patient is having difficulty breathing and that she gave herself an epinephrine auto-injection after being stung. When you arrive the patient is sitting up. Your general impression is that the patient is a young woman, about 28 years old, who is pale, sweating, and wheezing. She has blotches and hives on her neck and arms and her face looks swollen.

This patient is a high priority as her respiratory and circulatory systems are compromised. She is in anaphylactic shock. Her husband helped her with the epinephrine auto-injector, which was prescribed to her after the last time she was stung. The date on the injector indicates that it has not expired, and the syringe has been emptied.

Initial Assessment

Recording time
0 minutes

Appearance
Pale, sweaty, and unstable

Level of consciousness
Alert

Airway
Open

Vital Signs

Pulse rate/quality
140 beats/min, regular, weak

Blood pressure
80/40 mm Hg

Respiratory rate/depth
30 breaths/min, wheezing, shallow, and labored

Question 1: What is an antibody?

Question 2: What is an immune response?

Question 3: Describe the two general types of immune response.

essential for formation of mature blood cells. The bone marrow produces B lymphocytes.

In secondary lymphoid tissues, mature immune cells interact with invaders and initiate a response. Secondary tissues are divided into encapsulated tissues and unencapsulated diffuse lymphoid tissues. The <u>encapsulated lymphoid tissues</u> consist of the spleen and the lymph nodes. A <u>lymph node</u> (lymph gland) is a small structure that filters lymph and stores lymphocytes. Lymph nodes are concentrated in several areas of the body, such as the axillae, groin, and neck. The <u>spleen</u> is located on the left side of the body posterior and lateral to the stomach (left upper quadrant). This organ monitors the blood, destroys worn out red blood cells, and traps foreign invaders.

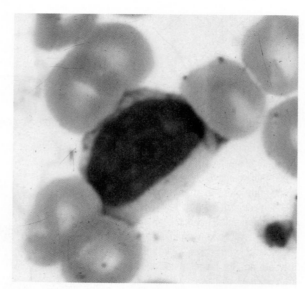

Figure 7-2 Structure of mature lymphocyte in the peripheral blood (original magnification, × 1,000).

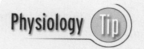

Antibodies are proteins secreted by lymphocytes that bind antigens and make them more visible to the immune system. Cytokines are protein messengers released by one cell that affect the growth or activity of another cell.

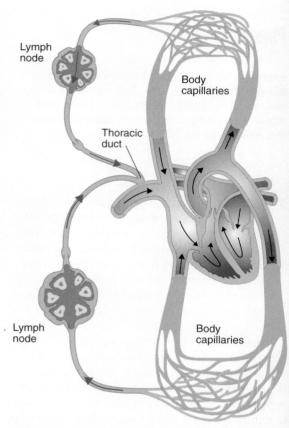

Figure 7-3 The interrelationship of the lymphatic system and the circulatory system. Blood fluid passes out of the arteries in the upper and lower parts of the body. It enters a system of lymphatic ducts that arise in the tissues. The fluid, called lymph, passes through lymph nodes and on the right side makes its way back to the general circulation via the thoracic duct. Lymph vessels from the left upper quadrant join the thoracic duct and empty into the left subclavian vein. Lymph vessels from the right upper quadrant join together to form the right lymphatic duct, which empties into the right subclavian vein.

The remainder of the tissues of the lymphatic system, called **diffuse lymphoid tissues**, are scattered throughout the body.

Lymph is a thin, watery fluid that bathes the tissues of the body. It circulates through lymph vessels and is filtered in lymph nodes. Lymphatic capillaries unite to form lymph vessels. The lymphatic vessels eventually coalesce and empty their contents into the central venous circulation. The majority of lymph empties into the superior vena cava via the thoracic duct, located on the left side of the thorax. The remaining lymph enters the right subclavian vein via three or four lymphatic ducts. The exact number of ducts varies from person to person (▶ **Figure 7-3**).

Clusters of lymphoid tissue are associated with the skin and the respiratory, urinary, gastrointestinal, and reproductive tracts. These tissues contain immune cells that are in a position to intercept pathogens before they get into the general circulation. All of these are collectively termed **mucosal-associated lymphoid tissue (MALT)**. The tonsils

are perhaps the best known type of MALT. Unencapsulated lymphoid tissue is particularly prominent in the gastrointestinal tract (▶ **Figure 7-4**). Called the **gut-associated lymphoid tissue (GALT)**, this tissue lies just under the inner lining of the esophagus and intestines.

The primary cells of the immune system are the white blood cells, or **leukocytes**. ▶ **Table 7-1** provides a summary of the white blood cells. There are five general types:

1. Basophils and mast cells – **Basophils** in the blood and **mast cells** in the tissues contain granules of histamine and other substances that are released during inflammatory and

allergic responses. Basophils account for less than 1% of the leukocytes but are essential to nonspecific immune response to inflammation due to their role in releasing histamine and chemicals that dilate blood vessels. Mast

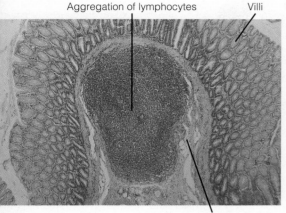

Aggregation of lymphocytes   Villi

Loose connective tissue

Figure 7-4 Lymphoid tissue. The loose connective tissue beneath the lining of the large intestine and other sites is often packed with lymphocytes that have proliferated in response to invading bacteria.

cells resemble basophils but do not circulate in the blood. They are found in the connective tissues, beneath the skin, in the gastrointestinal mucosa, and in the mucosal membranes of the respiratory system.

2. Eosinophils – <u>Eosinophils</u> are associated with parasitism and may release substances that damage or kill parasitic invaders. They also play a major role in mediating the allergic response. They account for 1% to 3% of the

Physiology Tip

Lymph nodes filter infection-causing organisms and other foreign matter from the blood. Sometime during the course of certain kinds of infections, the nodes become swollen and tender. This may indicate not only that an infection is present, but also that the body is utilizing its normal defense mechanisms to fight the invader.

Table 7-1
Summary of Blood Cells

Name	Description	Concentration (Number of Cells/mm^3)	Life Span	Function
Red blood cells (RBCs)	Biconcave disk; no nucleus	4–6 million	120 days	Transports oxygen and carbon dioxide
White blood cells				
Neutrophil	Approximately twice the size of RBCs; multilobed nucleus; clear-staining cytoplasm	3,000–7,000	6 hours to a few days	Phagocytizes bacteria
Eosinophil	Approximately same size as neutrophil; large pink-stained granules; bilobed nucleus	100–400	8–12 days	Phagocytizes antigen-antibody complex; attacks parasites
Basophil	Slightly smaller than neutrophil; contains large, purple cytoplasmic granules; bilobed nucleus	20–50	Few hours to a few days	Releases histamine during inflammation
Monocyte	Larger than neutrophil; cytoplasm grayish-blue; no cytoplasmic granules; U- or kidney-shaped nucleus	100–700	Lasts many months	Phagocytizes bacteria, dead cells, and cellular debris
Lymphocyte	Slightly smaller than neutrophil; large, relatively round nucleus that fills the cell	1,500–3,000	Can persist many years	Involved in immune protection, either attacking cells directly or producing antibodies
Platelets	Fragments of megakaryocytes; appear as small dark-staining nucleus	250,000	5–10 days	Play several key roles in blood clotting

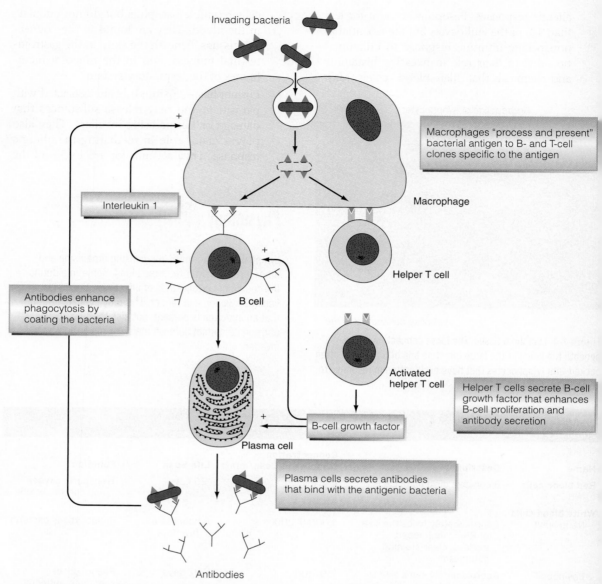

Invading bacteria

Macrophages "process and present" bacterial antigen to B- and T-cell clones specific to the antigen

Macrophage

Interleukin 1

Helper T cell

Antibodies enhance phagocytosis by coating the bacteria

B cell

Activated helper T cell

Helper T cells secrete B-cell growth factor that enhances B-cell proliferation and antibody secretion

B-cell growth factor

Plasma cell

Plasma cells secrete antibodies that bind with the antigenic bacteria

Antibodies

Figure 7-5 The role of the macrophage in immunity. Macrophages "present" antigen to B cells and helper T cells. They also phagocytize antibody-coated bacteria.

leukocytes and release chemoactive substances that can result in severe bronchospasm.

3. Neutrophils – <u>Neutrophils</u> are the most abundant white blood cell, accounting for approximately 55% to 70% of the leukocytes. They have a segmented nucleus and are often called <u>polymorphonuclear</u> leukocytes, or "polys." They are responsible in large part for the body's protection against infection and are the principle part of the first response to foreign body invasion. They are readily attracted by foreign antigens and destroy them by engulfing and digesting them. This process of engulfing a foreign substance is known as <u>phagocytosis</u> (▲ Figure 7-5).

4. Monocytes and macrophages – <u>Monocytes</u> are the precursors of macrophages. Monocytes mature in the blood during their first 24 hours and then travel to the tissues where they will differentiate into <u>macrophages</u>. Monocytes and macrophages are one of the first lines of defense in the inflammatory process. Macrophages function primarily as scavengers for the tissues.

5. Lymphocytes – <u>Lymphocytes</u> and their derivatives mediate the acquired immune

Physiology Tip

Macrophages play a major role in acquired immunity. When they ingest molecular or cellular substances and digest them, antigen fragments are processed and inserted into the macrophage membrane. This makes the antigen visible to other immune cells. Immune cells that process antigens in this fashion are called <u>antigen-presenting cells</u>.

Physiology Tip

Vaccinations using killed or weakened viruses stimulate the body's immune system to actively form antibodies, preventing the actual disease from ever occurring. This is a form of active acquired immunity.

Patients who are exposed to some forms of hepatitis are given an injection of gamma-globulin, a combination of antibodies. This produces a temporary boost in the immune system's ability to prevent actual infection by the invading pathogen. Gamma-globulin administration is a form of passive acquired immunity.

response. Most lymphocytes are found in the lymphoid tissues, although many are found in circulating lymph and blood as well. There are two basic types: B lymphocytes and T lymphocytes.

Characteristics of the Immune Response

There are two general types of immune response: native and acquired. The native and acquired immune responses protect us from potentially infectious agents (eg, viruses, bacteria) and foreign substances that have gained access to our body through the skin or the lining of our internal organs.

<u>Native immunity</u>, which is also referred to as natural or innate immunity, is a nonspecific cellular and humoral (antibody) response that operates as the first line of defense against pathogens. Most native immunity is associated with the initial inflammatory response (discussed in Chapter 8).

<u>Acquired immunity</u>, also referred to as adaptive immunity, is a highly specific, inducible, discriminatory, and unforgetting method by which armies of cells respond to an immune stimulant. <u>Active acquired immunity</u> occurs as a result of exposure of the body to a foreign substance or disease and is associated with antibody production to help prevent recurrence. <u>Passive acquired immunity</u> is the receipt of preformed antibodies to fight or prevent an infection. Typically passive acquired immunity lasts for a much shorter period of time than active acquired immunity. Examples include transplacental transmission of maternal antibodies, which protect newborn infants until their own immune system matures sufficiently to take over, and injection of immunoglobulin (a concentrated form of antibodies obtained from donors).

The primary, or <u>initial immune response</u>, takes place during the first exposure to a foreign substance.

Medication Tip

Whenever you conduct a patient assessment, it is essential to obtain a SAMPLE history. The "A" in SAMPLE represents "allergies." It is not uncommon to find that patients are allergic to medications such as penicillin or sulfa drugs. Often these patients are aware of their allergies because they have previously had very serious reactions to the medications. Another way that patients experience their first reaction to a medication is in the dentist office where they have a reaction to novocaine. These same patients are often allergic to other "caine" drugs, such as lidocaine, which may be used to manage frequent and/or multifocal premature ventricular contractions. For this reason it is always a good idea not only to ask patients if they are allergic to any medications, but also to inquire whether they have ever experienced a reaction to a shot during a dental office visit. You should also ask them about the reaction they had because some patients confuse the side effects of a drug (ie, nausea/vomiting) with a severe allergic reaction. Is it possible that they had an allergic reaction to the preservative in the vial of novocaine as opposed to the medication itself?

It may or may not result in clinical symptoms. Sometimes, the initial response of the body is to produce an antibody that causes symptoms on subsequent exposures. The secondary, or <u>amnestic immune response</u>, occurs upon repeat exposure to a foreign substance. The body has already developed a "memory" for that substance and on re-exposure a reaction occurs. The activation of B cells by an antigen is illustrated in ▶ **Figure 7-6.**

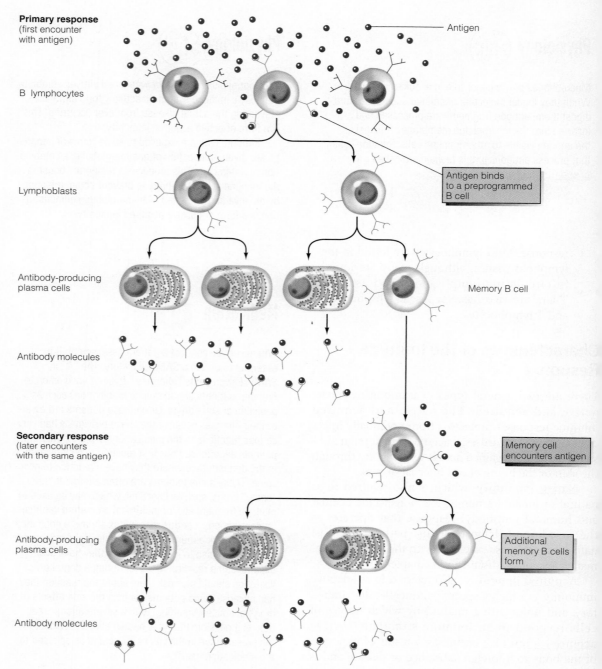

Primary response
(first encounter
with antigen)

Antigen

B lymphocytes

Antigen binds
to a preprogrammed
B cell

Lymphoblasts

Antibody-producing
plasma cells

Memory B cell

Antibody molecules

Secondary response
(later encounters
with the same antigen)

Memory cell
encounters antigen

Antibody-producing
plasma cells

Additional
memory B cells
form

Antibody molecules

Figure 7-6 B-cell activation. Immunocompetent B cells are stimulated by the presence of an antigen, producing an intermediate cell, the lymphoblast. The lymphoblasts divide, producing plasma cells and some memory T cells. Memory T cells respond to subsequent antigen encroachment, yielding a rapid, secondary response.

Immunity may be either humoral or cell mediated. In **humoral immunity**, antibodies are produced by B-cell lymphocytes. Antibodies react with a specific antigen (a foreign substance). In **cell-mediated immunity**, T-cell lymphocytes recognize antigens and either secrete substances (cytokines) that attract other cells or become cytotoxic ("killer") cells and kill infected or abnormal cells (▶ Figure 7-7).

Induction of the Immune Response

The beginning or induction phase of the immune response occurs when a part of the immune system recognizes an **antigen**—any foreign substance. Antigens may be either **immunogenic** (they elicit an immune response) or **nonimmunogenic** (do not elicit an immune response). An antibody binds a

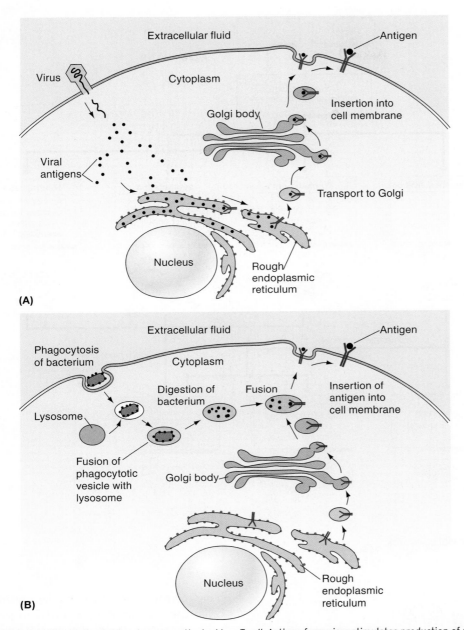

Figure 7-7 Cell-mediated immunity. **A.** Virus becomes attached to a T cell. Antigen from virus stimulates production of specific antigen, which is inserted onto cell membrane. **B.** Bacterium is digested by T lymphocyte, and antigen is presented on cell membrane.

specific antigen so that the complex can attach itself to specialized immune cells that either ingest the complex to destroy it or release biologic mediators such as histamine to induce an allergic/inflammatory response. The specific features of the antigen-antibody interaction depend on the foreign substance involved (▶ **Figure 7-8**)

An <u>immunogen</u> is an antigen that activates immune cells to generate an immune response against itself. Thus, an immunogen is an antigen, but an antigen is not necessarily an immunogen. A <u>hapten</u> is a substance that normally does not stimulate an immune response but that can be combined with an antigen and, at a later time, initiate a specific antibody response on its own.

Humoral Immune Response

B Lymphocytes

The humoral immune response occurs due to antibodies, which are made by <u>B lymphocytes</u> or B cells. Like all the blood cells, B cells are born in the

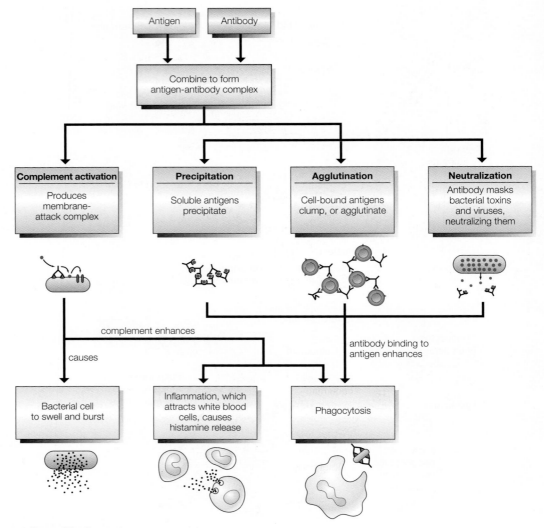

Figure 7-8 How antibodies work.

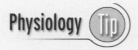

Did you ever wonder how the human body distinguishes between foreign substances and its own cells and tissues? The <u>major histocompatibility complex (MHC)</u> is a group of genes located on a single chromosome. The MHC permits an individual who is capable of generating an immune response to distinguish *self* from what is foreign, or *non-self*. The <u>human leukocyte antigen (HLA) gene complex</u> is the human MHC and is present in all nucleated human cells. It codes for numerous antigens that are unique to an individual. When the immune system "sees" these particular antigens, it recognizes them as "self," and no immune response occurs.

bone marrow, where they are descended from ster cells. Current thinking, referred to as the <u>clona selection theory</u>, holds that each B cell makes anti bodies that have only one type of antigen bindin region and, therefore, are specific for a specific anti gen, known as its <u>cognate antigen</u>. The antibodie are on the surface of B cells and are thus able to rec ognize the presence of their cognate antigens.

When a B cell recognizes the cognate antigen, proliferates to make more identical B cells, whic can make antibodies that recognize the same anti gen. In order for B cells to produce antibodies, the must first be activated. The most common way thi occurs is via <u>helper T cells</u>:

1. A macrophage engulfs the antigen via phago cytosis. It digests the antigen, pushing parti cles of antigen to the cell surface. Here, the

Table 7-2
Summary of Blood Types

Blood Type	Antigens on Plasma Membranes of RBCs	Antibodies in Blood	Safe to Transfuse To	From
A	A	b*	A, AB	A, O
B	B	a	B, AB	B, O
AB	A + B	—	AB	A, B, AB, O
O	—	a + b	A, B, AB, O	O

*Lowercase b indicates antibody to B antigen.

antigen interacts with the B cell and a helper T cell.

2. The antigen binds to both the B cell and the helper T cell, activating both.

3. The activated helper T cell secretes a substance, called a lymphokine, which stimulates the B cells to produce a clone. A clone is a group of identical cells formed from the same parent cell. The clone comprises two types of identical cells that have different functions: the plasma cells and the memory cells. Plasma cells make the antibodies, and memory cells "remember" the initial encounter with the antigen (▶ Figure 7-10).

Immunoglobulins

The antibodies secreted by B cells are called immunoglobulins. Chemically, they are Y-shaped proteins that consist of several regions, including a region that binds only a specific antigen. The basic antibody molecule has four chains linked into a Y-shape. Each side of the Y is identical, with one light chain attached to one heavy chain (▶ Figure 7-11). The two arms, or Fab regions, contain antigen-binding sites. The stem of the Y-shaped molecule is the Fc region and deter-

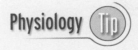
mines to which of the five immunoglobin classes an antibody belongs (▶ Figure 7-12). This text will use the terms immunoglobulins and antibodies interchangeably, unless otherwise stated.

Most antibodies are found in the plasma, where they make up about 20% of the plasma proteins in a healthy individual. Antibodies make antigens more visible to the immune system in three ways:

1. By acting as opsonins – Opsoninization occurs when an antibody coats an antigen to facilitate its recognition by immune cells. Antibodies are not toxic by themselves, but

Physiology Tip

Rh factor is a red blood cell antigen present in about 85% of the population. Blood for transfusions must be classified for Rh factor as well as for ABO blood group to prevent possible incompatibility reactions. If an Rh-negative person receives Rh-positive blood, hemolysis (rupture of red blood cells) and anemia may result (▼ **Figure 7-9**).

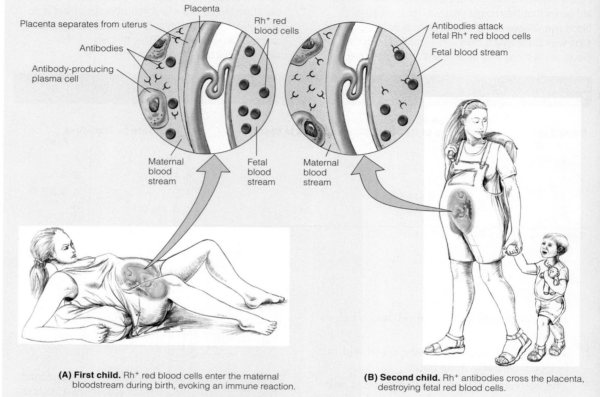

(A) First child. Rh⁺ red blood cells enter the maternal bloodstream during birth, evoking an immune reaction.

(B) Second child. Rh⁺ antibodies cross the placenta, destroying fetal red blood cells.

Figure 7-9 The Rh factor and pregnancy. **A.** Rh-positive cells from the fetus may enter the mother's blood at birth. If the mother is Rh-negative, her immune system responds, producing antibodies to the Rh-positive red blood cells and destroying them. **B.** Problems arise if the mother becomes pregnant again and has another Rh-positive baby. If the mother was not treated the first time, antibodies to Rh-positive red blood cells cross the placenta and destroy fetal red blood cells.

they label antigens so that other immune cells will attack them.

2. By making antigens clump (precipitation) – Antibodies cause antigens to clump for easier phagocytosis.

3. By inactivating bacterial toxins – Antibodies bind to and inactivate some toxins produced by bacteria. Macrophages can then ingest and destroy the inactivated toxins.

Antibodies are divided into five general classes of immunoglobulins-IgG, IgA, IgM, IgE, and IgD:

1. IgG – the most common, accounting for 75% of the antibodies in the blood. IgG is also found in the lymph, synovial fluid, peritoneal fluid, cerebrospinal fluid, and breast milk. It is the only immunoglobulin that crosses the placenta, giving infants immunity in the first few months of life.

Physiology (Tip)

Monoclonal antibodies are immunoglobulins secreted by a single clone of antibody-producing cells, either in vivo or in vitro. Such antibodies are specific for a particular antigen. These are used in diagnostic testing as well as therapeutically. Monoclonal antibodies to digoxin may be lifesaving in cases of severe intoxication or overdose.

2. IgA – accounts for 15% of the antibodies in the blood. Also found in tears, saliva, respiratory tract secretions, and the stomach. It combines with a protein in the mucosa and defends body surfaces against invading microorganisms.

3. IgM – accounts for 5% to 10% of the antibodies in the blood and is the dominant antibody in ABO incompatibilities. IgM is the initial antibody formed in most infections.

4. IgE – accounts for less than 1% of the antibodies in the blood and is associated with allergic reactions. When mast cell receptors combine with IgE and antigen, the mast cells degranulate and release chemical mediators such as histamine.

5. IgD – accounts for less than 1% of the antibodies in the blood. The physiologic role of IgD is unclear.

Cell-Mediated Immune Response

The cell-mediated immune response primarily involves T cells. T cells contribute to the immune defenses in two major ways. Some help regulate the complex workings of the immune system, while others are cytotoxic and directly contact infected cells and destroy them. There are four subgroups of T cells:

1. **Killer T cells** destroy the antigen; these are also called cytotoxic T cells. Cytotoxic T cells help rid the body of cells that have been infected by viruses as well as cells that have been transformed by cancer. They are also responsible for the rejection of tissue and organ grafts.

2. **Helper T cells** activate many immune cells, including B cells and other T cells (also called T4 or CD4$^+$ cells).

3. **Suppressor T cells** (also called T8 or CD8$^+$ cells) suppress the activity of other lymphocytes so they do not destroy normal tissue.

4. **Memory T cells** remember the reaction for the next time it is needed.

During the cell-mediated response, macrophages ingest pathogens. They digest the pathogen, releasing small particles of antigen. The antigen pushes its way to the macrophage surface where it is recognized by specific T cells. Other T cells, such as helper T cells and killer T cells, bind to the antigen and macrophage, and the invader is destroyed.

Cellular Interactions in the Immune Response

There are remarkable similarities in how the body responds to different kinds of immune challenges. The details depend on the particular challenge, but

---

Case Study

Case Study, Part 2

You lay the patient down and elevate her legs while your partner administers high-flow oxygen by nonrebreathing mask. The patient tells you that her tongue and throat feel swollen and she has chest tightness. Her lung sounds are diminished in the bases and wheezing is audible. A closer look reveals hives on her back, chest, abdomen, and extremities. The stinger was removed by her husband. The SpO2 reading is 90%, and electrocardiogram shows sinus tachycardia at 140 beats/min. She is going to need more epinephrine, IV fluids, and rapid transport to the hospital. The last time she was stung was 2 years ago, and she nearly died.

Focused Physical Assessment

Recording time
4 minutes

Signs and symptoms
Swollen tongue
Diminished lung sounds and wheezing
Head-to-toe angioedema (hives)

Diagnostic Tools

Electrocardiogram
Sinus tachycardia at 140 beats/min

SpO2
90%

Question 4: What are the possible routes by which an antigen may enter the body?

Question 5: What are the general classes of antibodies, and which one is associated with allergic reactions?

CASE STUDY

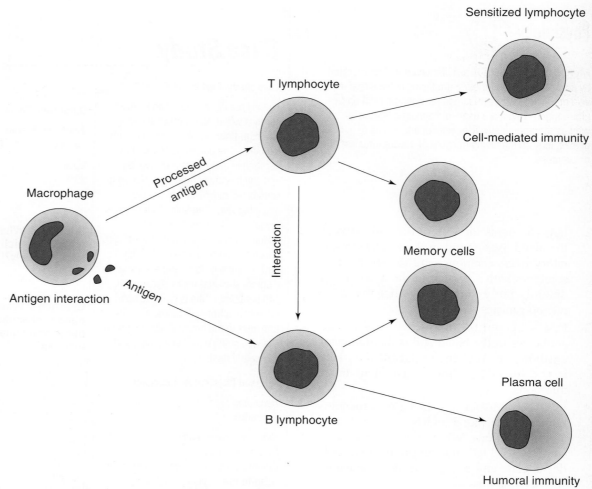

Figure 7-10 Interaction of cell-mediated and humoral immunity.

the basic pattern is the same. The innate response starts first and is then reinforced by the more specific acquired response. The two pathways are interconnected. Consider what happens when bacteria enter the body:

- If the bacteria are not encapsulated, macrophages begin to ingest them immediately. If the bacteria are encapsulated, antibodies (opsonins) must coat the capsule before they can be ingested by phagocytes.
- Components of the cell wall activate the complement system. Some components of the activated complement system, termed <u>**chemotaxins**</u>, attract leukocytes from the circulation to help fight the infection.
- The complement cascade ends in the formation of a set of proteins called the <u>**membrane attack complex (MAC)**</u>. These molecules

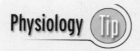

Cell-mediated immunity is responsible for <u>delayed hypersensitivity reactions</u>, such as those seen with poison ivy. The patient is exposed to an antigen and a reaction develops several hours later.

insert themselves into the bacterial membrane, leading to weakened areas in the membrane.

- Ions and water enter the cell through the weakened areas, leading to lysis of the bacterium. This is a chemical process and does not involve immune cells.
- If antibodies to the bacteria are already in the body, they will help the innate response by

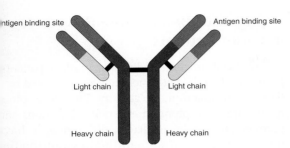

Figure 7-11 Structure of an immunoglobulin molecule.

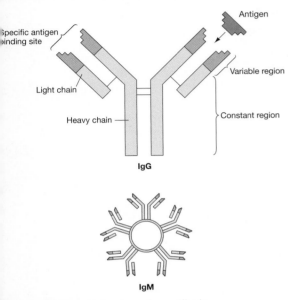

Figure 7-12 General structure of an antibody.

acting as opsonins and neutralizing bacterial toxins.

- Although it often takes several days, memory B cells attracted to the infection site will be activated if they encounter an antigen they recognize.
- If the infection is new to the body (preexisting antibodies are not present), B cells will be activated. Combined with helper T cells and cytokine release, antibodies are produced and memory B and T cells are formed.

Fetal and Neonatal Immune Function

Fetal immunity is a passive acquired immunity and is derived primarily from maternal IgG and IgM antibodies. Following delivery, these antibodies persist until the neonate's own B cells take over. A substantial number of antibodies are also transferred through breast milk, which is one of many reasons why experts favor breast-feeding.

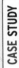
Case Study, Part 3

On scene, you were able to quickly start one IV and administer additional epinephrine. This is fortunate, considering the fact that vascular access can be very difficult on a patient in this condition. Rapid transport is begun and a second IV is started en route. You contact medical control to advise of the patient's condition and to obtain further treatment and medication orders. You receive additional orders and obtain another set of vital signs before proceeding. The patient is still pale and moist. The airway is still open, her lung sounds are not as diminished, but she is still wheezing. The hives are beginning to clear, and her blood pressure has not dropped any further.

Ongoing Assessment

Recording time
10 minutes

Mental status
Alert

Airway
Open

Skin signs
Pale and moist
Hives are improving.

Vital Signs

Pulse rate/quality
140 beats/ min, regular and weak

Blood pressure
80/40 mm Hg

Respiratory rate/depth
26 breaths/min, wheezing, labored

Diagnostic Tools

Electrocardiogram
Sinus tachycardia at 140 beats/min

SpO$_2$
98%

Question 6: Anaphylaxis occurs as a result of the release of what type of cells?

Question 7: What are the most common findings you can expect during an allergic response from the release of the type of cells in question 6?

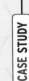
Case Study, Part 4

Completion of Case Study

Autoimmune reactions run a large gamut, from mild localized reactions to frank anaphylaxis with shock and death. Anaphylaxis involves IgE antigen interactions and includes the life-threatening cases involving hives, lip and throat swelling, wheezing, respiratory distress, and hypotension. Patients with acute anaphylactic reaction, exhibiting hypoperfusion and an altered mental status, should be treated with epinephrine. Management of the airway may include assisting ventilations or placing an endotracheal tube as needed. Management of circulation requires venous access and fluid resuscitation. Antihistamines such as diphenhydramine (Benadryl) are useful. Corticosteroids are a cornerstone of therapy, and vasopressors are useful for managing hypotension that does not respond to IV fluid therapy.

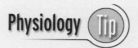

Physiology Tip

Autoimmune disease results when a breakdown in the mechanisms meant to preserve tolerance of "self" is severe enough to cause a pathologic condition. A common example is type 1 diabetes mellitus (insulin-dependent diabetes). Autoimmune attack occurs by production of antibodies against the insulin-producing beta cells of the pancreas.

Aging and the Immune Response in Older Patients

T- and B-cell function is deficient in older patients. Depressed lymphocyte function is accompanied by a decrease in macrophage activity. Therefore, older people are more prone to experience infections and recover slowly. In addition, older people have increased levels of autoantibodies (antibodies directed against the patient). This is one of the reasons why older people are prone to autoimmune disease.

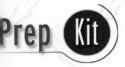

Chapter Summary

- The immune system includes all of the structures and processes that mount a defense against foreign substances and disease-causing agents. The body has three lines of defense: anatomic barriers, the inflammatory response, and the immune response.

- The lymphatic system is a network of capillaries, vessels, ducts, nodes, and organs that help to maintain the fluid environment of the body by producing lymph and transporting it through the body. The immune system has two anatomic components: the lymphoid tissues of the body and the cells that are responsible for the immune response.

- Lymphoid tissues are distributed throughout the body. The two primary lymphoid structures are the thymus gland and the bone marrow. Here cells involved in the immune response form and mature. Secondary lymphoid tissues are where mature immune cells interact with invaders and initiate a response. Secondary tissues are divided into encapsulated tissues and unencapsulated diffuse lymphoid tissues. The encapsulated lymphoid tissues are the spleen and the lymph nodes.

- Clusters of lymphoid tissue are associated with the skin and the respiratory, urinary, and reproductive tracts. These tissues contain immune cells that are in a position to intercept pathogens before they get into the general circulation. All of these tissues are collectively termed MALT.

- The primary cells of the immune system are the white blood cells, or leukocytes. There are five general types: basophils and mast cells, eosinophils, neutrophils, monocytes and macrophages, and lymphocytes. Each type of cell has a specific function during inflammation and activation of the immune system.

- There are two general types of immune response, native and acquired. Active acquired immunity occurs as a result of actually being exposed to a disease, then forming antibodies to help prevent recurrence. Passive acquired immunity is the receipt of preformed antibodies to fight or prevent an infection.

- Immunity may be either humoral or cell-mediated. In humoral immunity, antibodies are made by B-cell lymphocytes. Antibodies react with a specific antigen (a foreign substance). In cell-mediated immunity, T-cell lymphocytes recognize antigens and either secrete substances (cytokines) that attract other cells or become cytotoxic (killer) cells and kill infected or abnormal cells.

- The MHC is a group of genes located on a single chromosome. The MHC permits an individual who is capable of generating an immune response to distinguish self from what is foreign, or non-self. Red blood cells lack nuclei and thus, an MHC complex. To be recognized as self, the ABO blood group antigens and the Rh antigens evolved.

- The humoral immune response occurs due to antibodies, which are made by B lymphocytes or B cells. B cells are born in the bone marrow, where they are descended from stem cells. Each B cell makes antibodies that have only one type of antigen-binding region and, therefore, are specific for a specific antigen, known as its cognate antigen.

- When a B cell recognizes the cognate antigen, it proliferates to make more identical B cells that can make antibodies that recognize the same antigen. In order for B cells to produce antibodies, they must first be activated. The most common way this occurs is via helper T cells.

- The antibodies secreted by B cells are called immunoglobulins. Chemically, they are Y-shaped proteins that consist of several regions, including a region that binds only a specific antigen. Antibodies make antigens more visible to the immune system in three ways: acting as opsonins, making antigens clump, and inactivating bacterial toxins. Antibodies are divided into five general classes of immunoglobulins: IgG, IgA, IgM, IgE, and IgD.

- The cell-mediated immune response primarily involves T cells. There are four subgroups of T cells: killer T cells, helper T cells, suppressor T cells, and memory T cells. During the cell-mediated response, macrophages ingest pathogens. They digest the pathogen, releasing small particles of antigen. The antigen pushes its way to the macrophage surface where it is recognized by specific T cells. Other T cells, such as helper T cells and killer T cells, bind to the antigen and macrophage, and the invader is destroyed.

- During an immune response the innate response starts first and is reinforced by the more specific acquired response. The two pathways are interconnected.

- Fetal immunity is derived primarily from maternal IgG and IgM antibodies. After delivery, these antibodies persist until the neonate's own B cells mature and develop their own antibodies. Maternal antibodies generally provide some immunity for the first 4 to 6 months after birth. The immune responses reach full strength by approximately age 5 months.

- T- and B-cell function is deficient in older people. Depressed lymphocyte function is accompanied by a decrease in macrophage activity. Therefore, older people are more prone to experiencing infections and recover slowly.

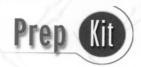

Vital Vocabulary

acquired immunity A highly specific, inducible, discriminatory, and permanent method by which literally armies of cells respond to an immune stimulant.

active acquired immunity The form of immunity that occurs as a result of being exposed to a disease; this exposure causes the body to form antibodies to help prevent recurrence.

amnestic immune response The reaction that occurs upon repeat exposure to a foreign substance.

antibodies Proteins secreted by certain immune cells that bind antigens to make them more visible to the immune system.

antigen A foreign substance recognized by the immune system.

antigen-presenting cells Cells that break down antigens and display their fragments on surface receptors to make them visible to the T lymphocytes. Macrophages are the primary antigen-presenting cells.

B lymphocytes Also called B cells, which develop in the bone marrow from stem cells.

basophils Approximately 1% of the leukocytes, they are essential to nonspecific immune response to inflammation due to their role in releasing histamine and other chemicals that dilate blood vessels.

bone marrow The specialized soft tissue that is found within the bone. The red bone marrow is essential for forming blood cells.

cell-mediated immunity Immune process by which T-cell lymphocytes recognize antigens and then secrete cytokines that attract other cells or become cytotoxic cells that kill the infected cells.

chemotaxins Components of the activated complement system that attract leukocytes from the circulation to help fight infections.

clonal selection theory The idea that each B cell makes antibodies that have only one type of antigen-binding region that is specific to a single type of antigen.

cognate antigen The specific antigen that binds to a specific region on the antibodies produced by B cells.

cytokines Protein messengers released by one cell that affects the growth of another cell.

delayed hypersensitivity reactions Immune reactions that occur several hours after exposure to an antigen.

diffuse lymphoid tissues All the secondary lymphoid tissues, with the exception of the spleen and lymph nodes, scattered throughout the body.

encapsulated lymphoid tissues Secondary lymphoid tissues consisting of the spleen and lymph nodes.

eosinophils Cells that make up approximately 1% to 3% of the leukocytes, which play a major role in allergic reactions and bronchoconstriction in an asthma attack.

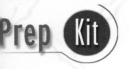

Fab regions The arms, which contain antigen-binding sites, of the Y-shaped immunoglobulin molecules.

Fc region The stem of the Y-shaped immunoglobulin molecule that determines the class of immunoglobin to which an antibody belongs.

gut-associated lymphoid tissue (GALT) The lymphoid tissue that lies under the inner lining of the esophagus and intestines.

hapten A substance that normally does not stimulate an immune response but can be combined with an antigen and at a later point initiate an antibody response.

helper T cells A type of T lymphocyte that is involved in both cell-mediated and antibody-mediated immune responses. It secretes cytokines that stimulate the B cells and other T cells.

human leukocyte antigen (HLA) gene complex The human MHC that is present in all nucleated human cells. It codes for numerous antigens that are unique to an individual.

humoral immunity The immunity that utilizes antibodies made by B-cell lymphocytes.

immune response The body's defense reaction to any substance that is recognized as foreign.

immune system The body system that includes all of the structures and processes designed to mount a defense against foreign substances and disease-causing agents.

immunogen An antigen that activates immune cells to generate an immune response against itself.

immunoglobulins Antibodies secreted by the B cells.

immunogenic Property of antigens indicating that they elicit an immune response.

initial immune response The reaction that takes place during the first exposure to a foreign substance.

leukocytes The white blood cells responsible for fighting off infection.

lymph A thin, watery fluid that bathes the tissues of the body.

lymph node A small structure that filters lymph and stores lymphocytes; also called lymph gland.

lymphocytes The white blood cells responsible for a large part of the body's immune protection.

lymphatic system A network of capillaries, vessels, ducts, nodes, and organs that help to maintain the fluid environment of the body by producing lymph and transporting it through the body.

macrophages Cells that developed from the monocytes and provide the body's first line of defense in the inflammatory process.

major histocompatibility complex (MHC) A group of genes located on a single chromosome that permits an organism that is capable of generating an immune response to distinguish a foreign substance from its own cells and tissues.

mast cells The cells that resemble basophils but do not circulate in the blood.

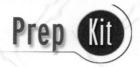

membrane attack complex (MAC) Molecules that insert themselves into the bacterial membrane, leading to weakened areas in the membrane.

memory cells One of the two types of cells in a clone that remember the initial encounter with the antigen.

monoclonal antibodies Immunoglobulins secreted by a single clone of antibody-producing cells, either in vivo or in culture.

monocytes The precursors of the macrophages, which are the body's first line of defense in the inflammatory process.

mucosal-associated lymphoid tissue (MALT) The lymphoid tissue associated with the skin and the respiratory, urinary, and reproductive traits as well as the tonsils.

native immunity A nonspecific cellular and humoral response that operates as the body's first line of defense against pathogens.

neutrophils Cells that make up approximately 55% to 70% of the leukocytes responsible in a large part for the body's protection against infection. They are readily attracted by foreign antigens and destroy them by phagocytosis.

nonimmunogenic Antigens that do not elicit an immune response.

opsoninization When an antibody coats an antigen to facilitate its recognition by immune cells.

passive acquired immunity The receipt of preformed antibodies to help fight and prevent recurrence of an infection.

phagocytosis When one cell eats or engulfs a foreign substance to destroy it.

plasma cells One of the two types of cells in a clone that make antibodies.

polymorphonuclear Possessing a nucleus consisting of several parts connected by fine strands.

primary/initial immune response A response that takes place during the first exposure to a foreign substance.

Rh factor A red blood cell antigen present in about 85% of people.

spleen The organ located in the left upper quadrant (LUQ) that monitors the blood and functions to destroy worn out red blood cells and trap foreign invaders.

thymus gland A bilobed gland situated below the thyroid gland and behind the sternum.

Case Study Answers

Question 1: What is an antibody?

Answer: Antibodies are protein substances formed by the body in response to antigens that have entered the body. Antibodies are secreted by certain immune cells that bind antigens and make them more visible to the immune system.

Question 2: What is an immune response?

Answer: When the body recognizes a foreign substance trying to invade the body, an immune response is set into motion. Protective cells recognize antigens or infections as they enter the body and destroy them to prevent and minimize harm to the body.

Question 3: Describe the two general types of immune response.

Answer: The two general types of immune response are native and acquired. Native immunity (also called natural or innate immunity) is a nonspecific cellular and humoral response that operates as the first line of defense against pathogens. Acquired immunity can be active or passive. Active acquired immunity occurs as a result of actually being exposed to a disease, then forming antibodies to help prevent recurrence. Passive acquired immunity is the receipt of preformed antibodies to fight or prevent an infection.

Question 4: What are the possible routes by which an antigen may enter the body?

Answer: Antigens can enter the body by inhalation, injection, absorption through the skin, or ingestion into the gastrointestinal tract.

Question 5: What are the general classes of antibodies, and which one is associated with allergic reactions?

Answer: Antibodies are divided into five general classes of immunoglobulins—IgG, IgA, IgM, IgE, and IgD. The immunoglobulin IgE accounts for less than 1% of the antibodies in the blood and is associated with allergic reactions and anaphylactic shock, which is the most serious of the reactions.

Question 6: Anaphylaxis occurs as a result of the release of what type of cells?

Answer: Anaphylaxis occurs as a result of the release of mediators such as histamine or other chemicals from mast cells. Mast cells are present in almost all organs and tissues, but the majority of these cells reside in the connective tissue, the skin, the respiratory tract, and the gastrointestinal tract.

Question 7: What are the most common findings you can expect during an allergic reaction from the release of the type of cells in question 6?

Answer: Because the majority of the mast cells are located in the connective tissue, skin, the gastrointestinal tract, and the respiratory tract, the most common findings you will see during an allergic response are hives, called urticaria, wheezing, and abdominal pain.

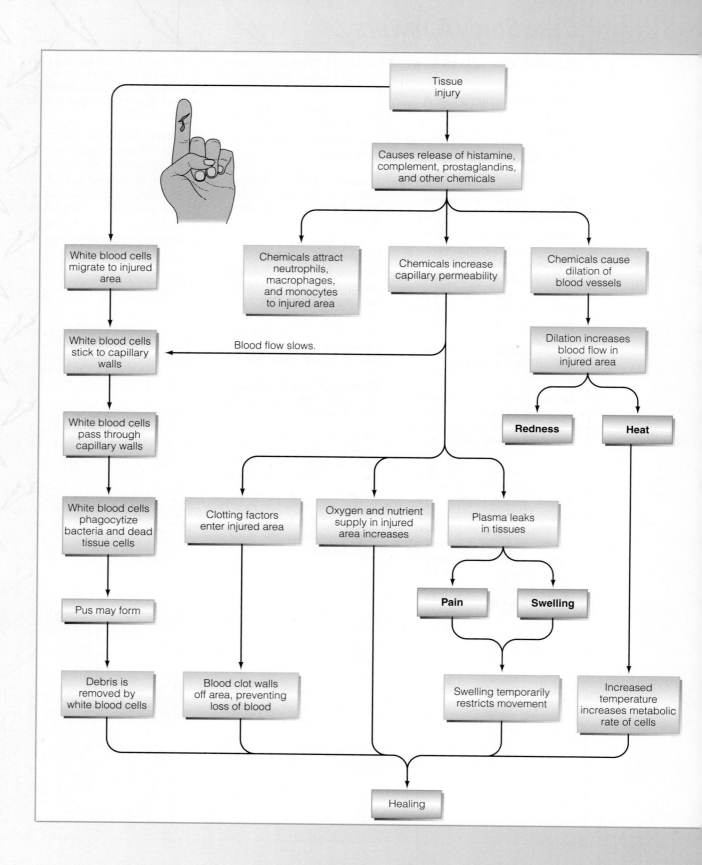

Inflammation 8

TECHNOLOGY

www.Paramedic.EMSzone.com

Online Chapter Pretest

Vocabulary Explorer

Anatomy Review

Web Links

Chapter FEATURES

Case Studies

Physiology Tips

Medication Tips

Paramedic Safety Tips

Special Needs Tips

Vital Vocabulary

Prep Kit

The Acute Inflammatory Response

The **inflammatory response** is the reaction of the body's tissues after irritation or injury that is characterized by pain, swelling, redness, and heat. It is triggered by any form of cellular injury, whether lethal or nonlethal. The two most common causes of inflammation are infection (eg, bacterial or viral) and injury.

The acute inflammatory response involves both vascular and cellular components. After transient arteriolar constriction, the arterioles dilate, allowing an influx of blood under increased pressure. This is termed **active hyperemia**. This increased intravascular pressure causes the blood vessel to expand, and like a balloon being inflated, the vessel walls become thinner. Pressure combined with increased vessel wall permeability leads to the fluid leaking into the interstitial spaces (**edema**). When enough fluid has leaked into the surrounding area (venules) and the intravascular pressure has been released, the vessel wall contracts and the outflow slows down, an action that contributes to **stasis of blood** in the capillaries.

Blood cells that participate in tissue inflammatory reactions are the white blood cells (leukocytes) and platelets. Specific cell types include neutrophils, monocytes (mast cells), lymphocytes, plasma cells, eosinophils, basophils, and activated platelets. Chemical mediators, primarily produced by the mast cells, account for the vascular and cellular events that occur during the acute inflammatory response. Cell-derived mediators include histamine, arachidonic acid derivatives, and cytokines (eg, interleukins, tumor necrosis factor).

Mast Cells

Mast cells play a major role in inflammation. During inflammation, they degranulate and release vasoactive amines and chemotactic factors. The major stimuli for degranulation of mast cells are physical injury (eg, trauma), chemical agents (eg, bacterial toxins), and immunologic substances (eg, interaction of an antigen and an IgE antibody). The most important **vasoactive amines** are **histamine** and **serotonin**. Both increase vascular permeability and cause vasodilation. They can also cause bronchoconstriction, nausea, and vomiting, which are familiar to EMT-Bs and paramedics from their experiences in the out-of-hospital setting. Because histamine is a preformed vasodepressor amine that is stored in mast cells, it can be released quickly, so its actions are seen early in the inflammatory response. Mast cells also synthesize chemotactic factors that

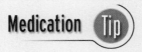

attract neutrophils and eosinophils; these are called neutrophil chemotactic factor and eosinophilic chemotactic factor, respectively.

Mast cells also synthesize leukotrienes and prostaglandins. **Leukotrienes** are a family of biologically active compounds derived from arachidonic acid. Leukotrienes are also sometimes referred to as **slow-reacting substances of anaphylaxis (SRS-A)**. The clinically important leukotrienes are LTB4 and the cysteinyl leukotrienes (CysLTs) because they participate in host defense reactions and pathophysiologic conditions that paramedics commonly see in the field, such as immediate hypersensitivity and inflammation. Leukotrienes have potent actions on many essential organs and systems, including the cardiovascular, pulmonary, immune and central nervous systems, and the gastrointestinal tract.

Leukotrienes are primarily endogenous mediators of inflammation. They contribute to the signs and symptoms seen in acute inflammatory responses. This includes responses resulting from the interaction of allergens with IgE antibodies on mast cells. The CysLTs are bronchoconstrictors. They also stimulate airway mucus secretion and are very potent at increasing the permeability of post-capillary venules—including those in the bronchial circulation—thereby causing plasma protein exudation (oozing out of the tissue) and edema. Recent evidence suggests that the CysLTs also promote eosinophil migration into the airways of animals and asthmatic patients. They may also increase bronchial hyperresponsiveness through an action on sensory nerves.

Prostaglandins are a group of about 20 lipids that are modified fatty acids attached to a five-member ring. Prostaglandins are also derived from arachidonic acid. They are found in many vertebrate tissues where they act as messengers involved in reproduction, the inflammatory response to infection, and pain. Aspirin and nonsteroidal antinflammatory drugs (NSAIDs) inhibit prostaglandin synthesis, leading to reduced inflammation and pain.

Plasma Protein Systems

Plasma-derived mediators that modulate the inflammatory process are called plasma protein systems. These include the complement system, the clotting system, and the kinin system. The interaction of these systems is vital to a normal inflammatory response. Each system consists of a cascade of biochemical reactions such that, as one compound is produced, it catalyzes the formation of the next one. This cascade process can be visualized as knocking over a line of dominos.

1. The <u>complement system</u> is a group of plasma proteins that function in one of three ways: they attract white blood cells to sites of inflammation, activate white blood cells, and directly destroy cells. The central compound in this complement "cascade" is called C3. The C3 is produced by one of the two "complement pathways" (like two choices down an algorithm): the classic pathway and the alternate pathway. The <u>classic pathway</u> starts when an antigen-antibody complex binds to a complement component (called C1); activation of the classic pathway is dependent on the presence of antibodies. The <u>alternate pathway</u> can be triggered by bacterial toxins and does not need antibodies to be activated. The relationship between the complement system and mediators of inflammation is illustrated in ▶ Figure 8-1.

   Regardless of which pathway is taken, the main products are the same: C3b, the anaphylatoxins, and the membrane attack complex (MAC). <u>Anaphylatoxins</u> (referred to as C3a, C4a, and C5a) stimulate smooth-muscle contraction and increase vascular permeability. This is done by stimulating release of histamine from mast cells and platelets. <u>C3b</u> coats bacteria, making it easier for macrophages to engulf them. The membrane attack complex (MAC) is a set of complement proteins (C5b, C6, C7, C8, and C9) that bind to form a hollow tube, much like a short straw, that can puncture into the plasma membrane of a cell. Transmembrane channels are formed that allow ions, water, and other small molecules to pass through the pore; the cell cannot maintain osmolarity and dies.

2. The <u>coagulation system</u> is vital to the formation of blood clots in the body as well as facilitating repairs to the vascular tree. Inflammation triggers the coagulation cascade, a complex series of factors and chemical actions that result in the formation of fibrin. <u>Fibrin</u> is the protein that polymerizes (bonds) to form the fibrous component of a blood clot. However, coagulation factors are counterbalanced by a variety of inhibitors, so that the coagulation is restricted to one

---

Case Study

Case Study, Part 1

Your unit is dispatched to a call for a "sick person." From the dispatch information this call sounds routine, but when you arrive at the residence the call quickly becomes complicated. The patient is a diabetic who is morbidly obese, weighing over 400 lb. He is in no immediate distress, but he is unable to ambulate due to deep ulcers on both of his lower legs. Your partner calls for help with lifting assistance and you begin to assess the patient.

The patient tells you he is 47 years old and has a history of diabetes. His health aide called EMS for transport for evaluation of worsening cellulitis associated with the ulcers on his left lower leg. This morning the patient has a fever. He is alert and has tender legs; he is unable to ambulate or bear weight. Next, you take a set of vital signs while you are waiting for lifting assistance. Right now the patient's condition is stable, even though he is going to require hospitalization for the treatment of his fever, cellulitis, and ulcers.

Initial Assessment

Recording time
0 minutes

Appearance
No distress

Level of consciousness
Alert

Airway
Open

Vital Signs

Pulse rate/quality
82 beats/min, regular, strong

Blood pressure
144/78 mm Hg

Respiratory rate/depth
24 breaths/min, nonlabored

Question 1: What are the activators of the body's typical response to inflammation?

Question 2: Why is this patient experiencing fever?

Question 3: What is the role of plasma protein systems in the inflammatory response?

CASE STUDY

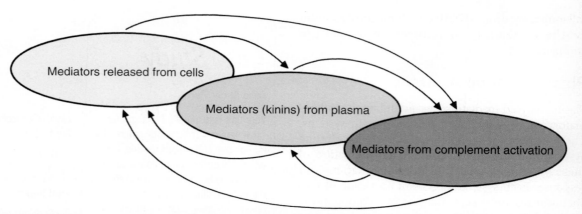

Figure 8-1 Interaction of mediators of inflammation. Activation of mediators from any source also leads to formation of mediators from other sources, which intensifies the inflammatory reaction.

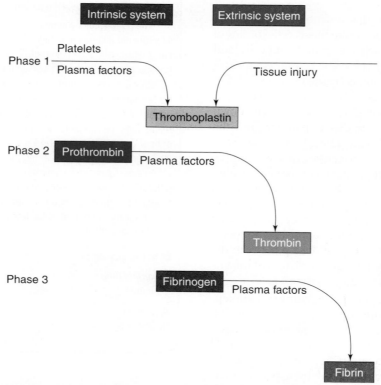

Figure 8-2 A simplified concept of the blood coagulation mechanism. In the intrinsic system, plasma factors (XII, XI, and IX) are activated, and they interact with factor VIII and platelets to yield intrinsic thromboplastin. In the extrinsic system, tissue injury yields extrinsic thromboplastin that reacts with a plasma factor (VII). Then the thromboplastin formed by either the intrinsic or extrinsic system interacts with additional components (factors V, X, and platelet phospholipids) to form the complex (prothrombin activator) that converts prothrombin into thrombin in the second phase. Thrombin converts fibrinogen into fibrin in the third phase.

area. Simultaneously, the **fibrinolysis cascade** is activated to dissolve the fibrin and create fibrin split products, which are fragments of a dissolving clot. A simplified concept of the blood coagulation mechanism is illustrated in ▲ **Figure 8-2**.

3. The **kinin** system leads to the formation of the vasoactive protein bradykinin from kallikrein. Kallikrein is an enzyme normally found in blood plasma, urine, and body tissue in an inactive state. When activated, it can dilate blood vessels, influence blood

pressure, modulate salt and water excretion of the kidneys, and influence cardiac remodeling after acute myocardial infarction. Bradykinin is a protein that increases vascular permeability, dilates blood vessels, contracts smooth muscle, and causes pain when injected into the skin.

The kinin system is initiated by the activation of **Hageman factor** (coagulation factor XII), a very important coagulation factor that links several major cascade systems. In addition to the kinin system, Hageman factor participates in the clotting, fibrinolytic, and complement cascades. The coagulation factors are listed in ▶ **Table 8-1**. Activators of Hageman factor include bacterial lipopolysaccharides and endotoxin.

Activated factor XII triggers the intrinsic clotting cascade, which occurs when the blood is exposed to collagen or other substances. For example, when a blood vessel is injured by a cut, the skin cells are damaged and the blood comes in contact with collagen. The extrinsic clotting cascade is activated by substances released from injured cells when tissue damage occurs. The process of blood clotting is illustrated in ▶ **Figure 8-3**.

Cellular Components of Inflammation

The goal of the cellular component of acute inflammation is for inflammatory cells (neutrophils) to arrive at the sites within tissue where they are needed. The steps of this process include an intravascular phase and an extravascular phase. During the intravascular phase, leukocytes move (marginate) to the sides of blood vessels and attach to the endothelial cells. During the extravascular phase, leukocytes travel to the site of inflammation and kill organisms.

Polymorphonuclear neutrophils (PMNs) are the primary effector cells in acute inflammation. Cellular events are as follows:

1. **Margination** – Loss of fluid from the blood vessels into the tissue causes the blood left in the vessels to have an increased viscosity. This increased viscosity slows the flow of blood and produces stasis. PMNs, which usually travel toward the center of the vessel, settle toward the sides of the vessel as the blood flow through the vessel slows down. As stasis develops, leukocytes also move (marginate) toward the sides of blood vessels, where they bump into the endothelial

cells and bind to them. Stress can lead to demargination of some white blood cells, which stimulates the bone marrow to produce more white blood cells, which increases the white blood cell count. The primary avenue for PMNs to travel to an inflamed or infected site is by margination, where they leak (an action termed *diapedesis*) through the vessel wall into the tissues.

2. **Activation** – Mediators of inflammation trigger the appearance of molecules known as selectins and integrins on the surfaces of endothelial cells and PMNs, respectively.

3. **Adhesion** – PMNs adhere to endothelial cells. This is mediated by selectins and integrins.

4. **Transmigration (diapedesis)** – The PMNs permeate through the vessel wall, moving into the interstitial space.

Case Study

Case Study, Part 2

You look at the patient's area of cellulitis as you begin the focused physical assessment. The bandages over the ulcers are clean and appear freshly dressed; there is no need to take them off. Just above the bandage on the left leg you see a large area of skin that appears red and edematous, and looks strangely like the skin of an orange. With gloves on you can feel that the area is hot to the touch compared with the other leg.

This patient is going to need antibiotics to treat the cellulitis. This treatment is not something you can provide in the prehospital setting. Your care will include safely moving the patient and keeping him comfortable. This can be complicated because of his weight.

The patient's SAMPLE history includes a new onset of fever this morning; he is allergic to sulfa drugs; he takes insulin in the morning and evening; his last glucose reading an hour ago was 160 mg/dL; he also takes blood pressure medication, a

diuretic, and blood thinner. He ate breakfast before he took the insulin.

Focused Physical Assessment

Recording time
10 minutes

Skin signs
Red, hot, edematous
Bandages are clean.

Vital Signs

Unchanged

Diagnostic Tools

Blood glucose level
160 mg/dL

Question 4: What is leukocytosis? Is it occurring with this patient?

Question 5: What are the cellular components of inflammation and what are their roles?

Table 8-1
Coagulation Factors

Factor Number	Name	Functions
I	Fibrinogen	Protein synthesized in liver; converted into fibrin in Stage 3
II	Prothrombin	Protein synthesized in liver (requires vitamin K); converted into thrombin in Stage 2
III	Tissue thromboplastin	Released from damaged tissue; required in extrinsic Stage 1
IV	Calcium ions	Required throughout entire clotting sequence
V	Proaccelerin (labile factor)	Protein synthesized in liver; required to form prothrombin activator in both intrinsic and extrinsic Stage 1
VII	Serum prothrombin conversion accelerator (stable factor, proconvertin)	Protein synthesized in liver (requires vitamin K); functions in extrinsic Stage 1
VIII	Antihemophilic factor (antihemophilic globulin)	Protein synthesized in liver; required for intrinsic Stage 1
IX	Plasma thromboplastin component	Protein synthesized in liver (requires vitamin K); required for intrinsic Stage 1
X	Stuart factor (Stuart-Prower factor)	Protein synthesized in liver (requires vitamin K); required to form prothrombin activator in both intrinsic and extrinsic Stage 1
XI	Plasma thromboplastin antecedent	Protein synthesized in liver; required for intrinsic Stage 1
XII	Hageman factor	Protein required for intrinsic Stage 1
XIII	Fibrin-stabilizing factor	Protein required to stabilize the fibrin strands in Stage 3

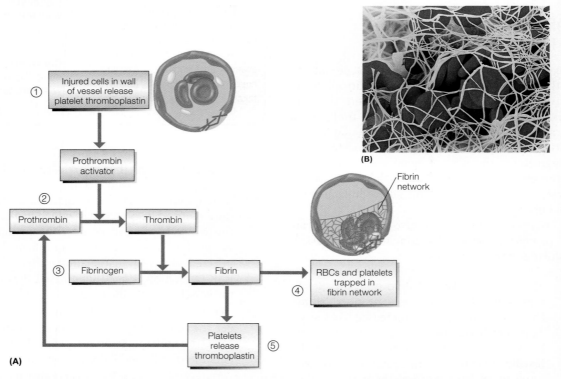

Figure 8-3 Blood clotting simplified. **A.** Injured cells in the walls of blood vessels release the chemical thromboplastin (1). Thromboplastin stimulates the conversion of prothrombin, found in the plasma, into thrombin (2). Thrombin, in turn, stimulates the conversion of the plasma protein fibrinogen into fibrin (3). The fibrin network captures red blood cells and platelets (4). Platelets in the blood clot release platelet thromboplastin (5), which converts additional plasma prothrombin into thrombin. Thrombin, in turn, stimulates the production of additional fibrin. **B.** A scanning electron micrograph of a fibrin clot that has already trapped platelets and red blood cells, plugging a leak in a vessel. The red blood cells are red and the fibrin network is turquoise.

5. <u>Chemotaxis</u> – PMNs move toward the site of inflammation in response to chemotactic factors that are released by bacteria or formed from activated complement, chemokines, or arachidonic acid derivatives (eg, leukotrienes) in response to cell injury.

The inflammatory response is illustrated in ▶ **Figure 8-4**.

<u>Monocytes</u> are a type of leukocyte that gives rise to many different types of cells, collectively known as the mononuclear phagocytic system. <u>Macrophages</u> are monocytes that have left the blood and entered into the tissues, thereby being transformed into larger phagocytic cells. Essentially, monocytes and macrophages are the same type of cell. When it is found in the blood, this cell is called a monocyte, and when in tissue it is called a macrophage.

Eosinophils contain granules of histamine and are involved in the allergic response. They are also part of the acute inflammatory response in a limited number of infections (eg, parasitic infections).

Cellular Products

<u>Cytokines</u> are products of cells that affect the function of other cells. Monocytes release <u>monokines</u>, and lymphocytes release <u>lymphokines</u>. Important categories of cytokines include:

1. <u>Interleukins</u> – IL-1 (interleukin-1) and IL-2 (interleukin-2) attract white blood cells to the sites of injury and bacterial invasion.

2. Lymphokines – stimulate leukocytes. <u>Macrophage-activating factor</u> stimulates macrophages to help engulf and destroy foreign substances. <u>Migration inhibitory factor</u> keeps white blood cells at the site of infection or injury until they can perform their designated task.

3. <u>Interferon</u> – produced by cells when they are invaded by viruses. Interferon is released into the bloodstream or intercellular fluid to induce healthy cells to manufacture an enzyme that counters the infection (▶ **Figure 8-5**).

Systemic Responses of Acute Inflammation

The degree of systemic response to acute inflammation depends on its severity. Common responses seen by the paramedic in the field include:

- Fever – White blood cells produce <u>pyrogens</u>, which are chemicals or proteins that travel to

the brain and affect the hypothalamus, and stimulate a rise in the body's core temperature.

- <u>Leukocytosis</u> – The normal body response to inflammation, regardless of the cause, is for the white blood cell count to be elevated. In bacterial infections, a significant portion of the white blood cells are neutrophils. One reason for this increased number of neutrophils is that the bone marrow is releasing more neutrophils and their precursors (bands). Some patients are so sick that they are unable to mount an effective leukocytosis. Leukocytosis is also a very common response to both physiologic and pathophysiologic stress. In some cases of severe sepsis, leukopenia (a lack of circulating white blood cells) can also be encountered. The main cause of the leukocytosis is demargination of white blood cells that have normally been "hanging around" on the vessel wall.

- Increase in circulating plasma proteins or acute-phase reactants; the most commonly

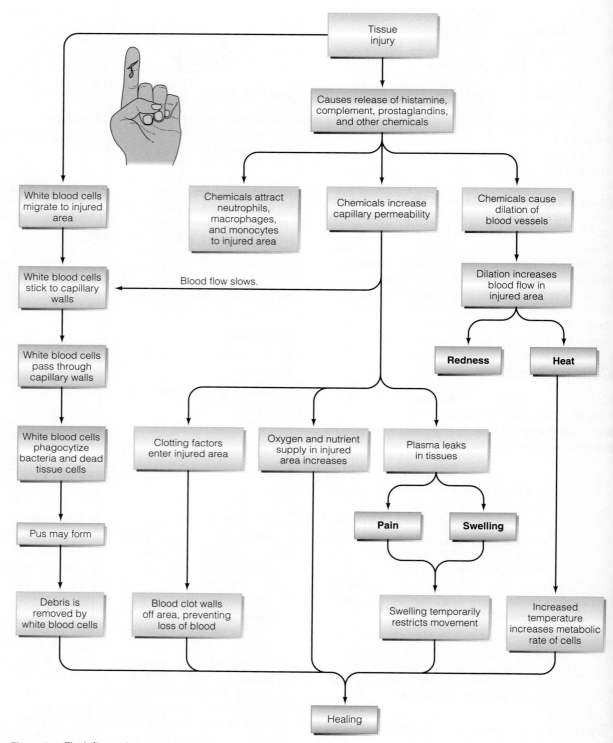

Figure 8-4 The inflammatory response.

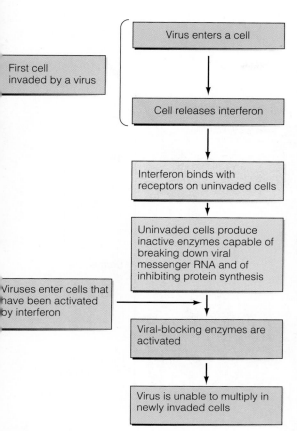

Figure 8-5 How interferon works. Interferon protects cells from viral infection.

Case Study

Case Study, Part 4

Completion of Case Study

Hyperglycemia is responsible for most of the long-term microvascular complications of diabetes, such as diabetic peripheral neuropathy, with resultant sensory deprivation that can impair the perception of trauma (eg, poorly fitting shoes, bumping into sharp objects). There is an increased risk of infection due to decreased cellular immunity caused by acute hyperglycemia and circulatory deficits caused by chronic hyperglycemia. Peripheral skin infections are common. Secondary infections from bacterial invasion occur in lesions, cracks, and ulcerations. Deep ulcers and ulcers associated with cellulitis may require hospitalization and may lead to toxic and permanent disability.

Signs and symptoms of cellulitis in the affected area include hot skin temperature and red skin that appears edematous, with texture similar to an orange. Systemic signs and symptoms can develop, especially in diabetic patients. These may include fever, chills, tachycardia, headache, hypotension, and altered mental status, yet many patients do not appear sick.

elevated protein in acute inflammation is C-reactive protein (CRP). It is not routinely measured during an acute infection or other form of inflammation. The most common use of high-sensitivity CRP measurements is in the ongoing management of persons at risk for heart attacks and strokes. Inflammation is a major component of both, and medical literature supports the concept that elevations of CRP identify persons who are at higher risk.

Chronic Inflammation Responses

Chronic inflammation responses are usually caused by an unsuccessful acute inflammatory response due to a foreign body, persistent infection, or antigen. They are associated with an infiltrate containing monocytes and lymphocytes, and usually involve tissue destruction and repair (or scar formation). The vascular events are similar to those that take place in acute inflammation but also include the growth of new blood vessels known as <u>angiogenesis</u>.

Injury Resolution and Repair

Normal wound healing involves four steps: repair of damaged tissue; removal of inflammatory debris; restoration of tissues to a normal state; and regeneration of cells. Healing after tissue injury or loss caused by inflammation depends on the type of cells, listed below, that make up the affected organ.

1. <u>Labile cells</u> divide continuously. Organs derived from these cells (eg, skin or intestinal mucosa) heal completely.

2. <u>Stable cells</u> are replaced by regeneration from remaining cells, which are stimulated to enter mitosis. Stable cells are found in the liver and kidney.

3. <u>Permanent cells</u> such as nerve cells and cardiac myocytes cannot be replaced. Scar tissue is laid down instead.

Healing by primary intention occurs in clean wounds with apposed margins (eg, a clean surgical wound). An illustration of the normal structure of the skin is illustrated in ▸ **Figure 8-6**.

Healing progresses in several stages:

1. Blood fills the defect and coagulates, forming a <u>scab</u>, which is a mesh-like structure composed of fibrin and fibronectin. If the inflammatory process was severe, tissue may be

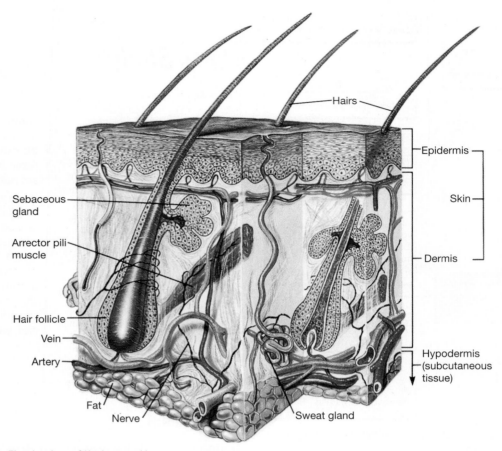

Figure 8-6 The structure of the human skin.

destroyed and require repair, as illustrated by the superficial necrosis shown in ▶ **Figure 8-7**.

2. Macrophages remove cellular debris and secrete growth factors. These stimulate angiogenesis and ingrowth of fibroblasts, leading to the formation of **granulation tissue**.

3. The epithelium regenerates, covering the surface defect.

4. Deposition of collagen results in **fibrous union**. By the end of the first week, 10% of the preoperative strength is regained.

5. **Scar maturation** occurs as collagen crosslinking takes place. By the end of 3 months, 80% of the normal tensile strength of the tissue has been restored.

Healing by secondary intention occurs in large gaping or infected wounds. Wounds that heal by secondary intention have a more pronounced and prolonged inflammatory phase causing the neutrophils to persist for days. They also have more abundant granulation tissue. Wound contraction is mediated by myofibroblasts, which help to draw the margins of the wound closer to one another as time passes.

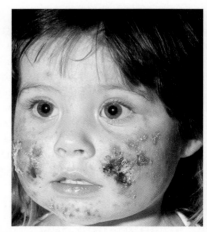

Figure 8-7 Acute inflammation of face with superficial necrosis of skin. Crusts of dried exudates (scabs) have formed on skin surface.

Factors that can lead to dysfunctional wound healing may be both local and systemic. Local factors include:

- Infection – when the body's healing efforts are diverted to fighting off the cause of the infection.

- Blood – an inadequate blood supply (as in diabetes) produces tissue hypoxia, which slows wound healing and may promote infection.
- Foreign bodies – when present in a wound, these stimulate acute and chronic inflammation, both of which interfere with wound healing.

Systemic factors that influence the healing of a patient's wounds include:

- Nutrition – poor nutritional intake leads to poor scar formation and suppression of the immune system.
- Hematologic abnormalities – proper wound healing requires the presence of adequate numbers of white blood cells. Patients who have impaired bone marrow stores of white blood cells are susceptible to infection and often heal slower.
- Systemic disease – both diabetes and acquired immunodeficiency syndrome (AIDS) affect the cells of the immune system, which plays a direct role in wound healing. In addition, there is an increased tendency for wound infection, which also interferes with normal healing. As mentioned earlier, diabetic patients often have an impaired circulation, especially in the lower extremities, which significantly slows the healing process and increases the likelihood of wound infection.
- Corticosteroid use – corticosteroids suppress the initial inflammatory response required for the proper formation of scar tissue. They also increase the risk of wound infection by slowing the immune system response.

Age and the Immune Response

Both newborns and geriatric patients often exhibit relative impairment of their immune systems, potentially slowing their inflammatory response. Thus, signs of inflammation are more subtle in these populations. In addition, wound healing often takes longer, especially in the geriatric patient. The immune system is not fully developed until the child is between 2 and 3 years of age. Therefore, investigation of a fever in younger children must be aggressive and thorough. Many experts recommend hospital admission for a temperature greater than 100.4°F in a child younger than 3 months.

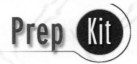

Chapter Summary

- The inflammatory response is a reaction of the tissues of the body to irritation or injury that is characterized by pain, swelling, redness, and heat. It is triggered by cellular injury. The two most common causes of inflammation are infection (eg, bacterial, viral) and physical agents (eg, tissue injury).

- The acute inflammatory response involves both vascular and cellular components. Blood cells that participate in tissue inflammatory reactions are the white blood cells (leukocytes). Chemical mediators account for the vascular and cellular events that occur during the acute inflammatory response. Cell-derived mediators include histamine, arachidonic acid derivatives, and cytokines (eg, interleukins, tumor necrosis factor).

- Mast cells play a major role in inflammation. They degranulate and release vasoactive amines and chemotactic factors. Mast cells also synthesize chemotactic factors, leukotrienes, and prostaglandins.

- Plasma protein systems are the plasma-derived mediators that modulate the inflammatory mediators. They include the complement system, the clotting system, and the kinin system. The interaction of these systems is vital to the normal inflammatory response. All three plasma protein systems are triggered by the activation of Hageman factor (coagulation factor XII).

- The goal of the cellular component of acute inflammation is for neutrophils to arrive at the sites within tissue where they are needed. The steps of this process involve an intravascular phase and an extravascular phase. During the intravascular phase, leukocytes marginate to the sides of blood vessels and attach to the endothelial cells. During the extravascular phase, leukocytes migrate to the site of inflammation and kill organisms.

- Cytokines are products of cells that affect the function of other cells. Major cytokines include the interleukins, lymphokines, and interferon.

- Systemic responses of the body to inflammation vary, depending on the stimulus. Typically, these include fever, leukocytosis, and increased levels of certain plasma proteins (acute phase reactants), especially C-reactive protein.

- Chronic inflammatory responses are usually caused by an unsuccessful acute inflammatory response after the invasion of a foreign body, persistent infection, or antigen. They are associated with an infiltrate containing monocytes and lymphocytes and usually are involved with tissue destruction and repair (or scar formation).

- Normal wound healing involves four steps: repair of damaged tissue; removal of inflammatory debris; restoration of tissues to a normal state; and regeneration of cells. Wounds may heal by either primary or secondary intention.

- Numerous factors (eg, infection, systemic disease) interfere with the normal response to inflammation. Those at extremes of age (eg, newborns, geriatric patients) have less effective inflammatory responses and wound healing ability.

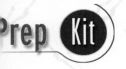

Prep Kit

Vital Vocabulary

Activation Mediators of inflammation that trigger the appearance of molecules known as selectins and integrins on the surfaces of endothelial cells.

Active hyperemia The dilation of arterioles after transient arteriolar constriction, which allows influx of blood under increased pressure.

Adhesion Holding together or uniting of two surfaces or parts, as in wound healing.

Alternate pathway A complement pathway that can directly convert C3 without the formation of C1.

Anaphylatoxins Part of the complement system consisting of C3a, C4a, and C5a, which stimulates smooth-muscle contraction and increased vascular permeability.

Angiogenesis The growth of new blood vessels.

C3b A complement component that coats bacteria, making it easier for macrophages to engulf the bacteria.

Chemotaxis The movement of additional white blood cells to an area of inflammation in response to the release of chemical mediators, such as neutrophils, injured tissue, and monocytes.

Classic pathway A complement pathway initiated by binding of an antigen-antibody complex to a complement component called C1.

Coagulation system The system that forms blood clots in the body and facilitates repairs to the vascular tree.

Complement system A group of plasma proteins whose function is to do one of three things: attract leukocytes to sites of inflammation; activate leukocytes; and directly destroy cells.

Cytokines Products of cells that affect the function of other cells; these hormonelike proteins regulate the intensity and duration of the immune response and mediate cell-cell communication.

Edema Collection of fluid into the perivascular space (the area surrounding a blood or lymph vessel).

Fibrin A whitish, filamentous protein formed by the action of thrombin on fibrinogen. Fibrin is the protein that polymerizes (bonds) to form the fibrous component of a blood clot.

Fibrinolysis cascade The breakdown of fibrin in blood clots, and the prevention of the polymerization of fibrin into new clots.

Fibrous union The result of deposition of collagen in the healing of a wound in the repair and restorative process.

Granulation tissue Type of tissue formed during the wound healing process from the ingrowth of fibroblasts.

Hageman factor Coagulation factor XII; an important coagulation factor that links several major cascade systems.

histamine A vasoactive amine that increases vascular permeability and causes vasodilation.

inflammatory response A reaction by tissues of the body to irritation or injury, characterized by pain, swelling, redness, and heat.

interferon Protein produced by cells in response to viral invasion. Interferon is released into the bloodstream or intercellular fluid to induce healthy cells to manufacture an enzyme that counters the infection.

interleukins Chemical substances that attract white blood cells to the sites of injury and bacterial invasion.

kinin A general term for a group of polypeptides that mediate inflammatory responses by stimulating visceral smooth muscle and relaxing vascular smooth muscle to produce vasodilation.

labile cells A type of cell that divides continuously and is found in the skin and intestinal mucosa; these cells heal more rapidly than other types of cells.

leukocytosis Elevation of the white blood cell count often due to inflammation.

leukotrienes Arachidonic acid metabolites that function as chemical mediators of inflammation.

lymphokines Cytokines released by lymphocytes, including many of the interleukins, gamma interferon, tumor necrosis factor beta, and chemokines.

macrophage-activating factor A cytokine that stimulates macrophages to help engulf and destroy foreign substances.

macrophages Monocytes that have left the blood, entered the tissues, and transformed into larger phagocytic cells.

margination Loss of fluid from the blood vessels into the tissue, causing the blood left in the vessels to have an increased viscosity, which in turn slows the flow of blood and produces stasis.

migration inhibitory factor A cytokine that keeps white blood cells at the site of infection or injury until they can perform their designated task.

monocytes Mononuclear phagocytic white blood cells derived from myeloid stem cells. They circulate in the bloodstream for about 24 hours and then move into tissues to mature into macrophages.

monokines Chemical mediators released by monocytes and macrophages during the immune response.

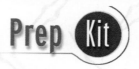

permanent cells Those cells that cannot be replaced, such as nerve cells and myocytes.

polymorphonuclear neutrophils (PMNs) A type of white blood cell formed by bone marrow tissue that possesses a nucleus consisting of several parts or lobes connected by fine strands; a variety of leukocyte.

prostaglandins A group of lipids that act as chemical messengers.

pyrogens Chemicals or proteins that travel to the brain and affect the hypothalamus, and stimulate a rise in the body's core temperature.

scab A meshwork of fibrin and fibronectin that develops over some wounds during healing.

scar maturation Phase of wound healing that occurs as collagen cross-linking takes place.

serotonin A vasoactive amine that increases vascular permeability to cause vasodilation.

slow-reacting substances of anaphylaxis (SRS-A) Biologically active compounds derived from arachidonic acid called leukotrienes.

stable cells Cells that are replaced through regeneration during wound healing.

stasis of blood Stagnation of blood in capillaries that occurs when capillary veins are dilated.

transmigration (diapedesis) The process by which bloo cells pass through capillary membranes into the tissues.

vasoactive amines Substances such as histamine and serotonin that increase vascular permeability.

Case Study Answers

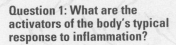

Question 1: What are the activators of the body's typical response to inflammation?

Answer: Typical activators of the acute inflammatory response include cellular injury and other microorganisms (eg, bacteria). The two most common causes are infection and tissue injury.

Question 2: Why is the patient experiencing fever?

Answer: Interleukin-1 will have attracted white blood cells to the site of the infection. Pyrogens produced by the white blood cells travel to the brain and initiate metabolic changes in the hypothalamic thermoregulatory center, causing a fever.

Question 3: What is the role of plasma protein systems in the inflammatory response?

Answer: Plasma protein systems include the complement system, the clotting system, and the kinin system. Each system consists of a flow of biochemical reactions such that as one compound is produced, it catalyzes the formation of the next one in a cascade.

Question 4: What is leukocytosis? Is it occurring with this patient?

Answer: Leukocytosis is the increased concentration of white blood cells in the blood. This is a normal response to inflammation in the body from a bacterial infection. Leukocytosis may or may not occur with cellulitis.

Question 5: What are the cellular components of inflammation and what are their roles?

Answer: The cellular components of inflammation include:

Phagocytes – engulf bacteria and foreign matter.

Polymorphonuclear neutrophils – destroy invading organisms, primarily bacteria.

Monocytes – produced in the bone marrow and through the process of phagocytosis enter tissues and are transformed into macrophages.

Macrophages – present antigens to helper T cells and polymorphonuclear neutrophils.

Eosinophils – produced in the bone marrow and destroy parasites, while also playing a major role in the pathogenesis of allergic reactions and asthma.

Question 6: What cellular products are involved in the inflammatory response and what are their roles?

Answer: The cellular products that are involved in the inflammatory response include:

Interleukin-1 and interleukin-2 – cytokines that attract white blood cells to the sites of injury and bacterial invasion.

Lymphokines – hormonelike peptide released by activated lymphocytes to mediate the immune response; a cytokine obtained by lymphocytes.

Macrophage-activating factor – stimulates macrophages to help engulf and destroy foreign substances.

Migration inhibitory factor – keeps white blood cells at the site of infection or injury until they can perform their mission.

Interferon – induces healthy cells to manufacture an enzyme that counters the infection.

Question 7: Why should hospitalization be considered right away for this patient?

Answer: Deep ulcers and ulcers associated with cellulitis may require hospitalization because they can lead to toxicity and permanent disability. Treatment will usually involve antibiotics and removal of inflammatory debris. In some advanced cases, the treatment may involve an amputation. The fact that this patient is a diabetic would increase that risk.

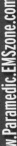

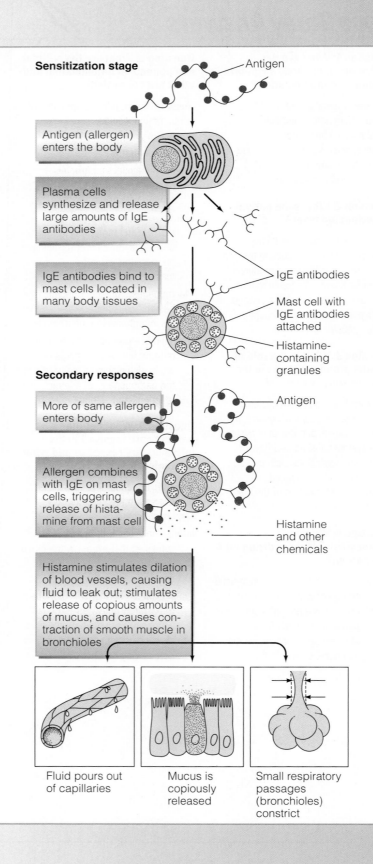

Sensitization stage

Antigen

Antigen (allergen) enters the body

Plasma cells synthesize and release large amounts of IgE antibodies

IgE antibodies bind to mast cells located in many body tissues

IgE antibodies

Mast cell with IgE antibodies attached

Histamine-containing granules

Secondary responses

More of same allergen enters body

Antigen

Allergen combines with IgE on mast cells, triggering release of histamine from mast cell

Histamine and other chemicals

Histamine stimulates dilation of blood vessels, causing fluid to leak out; stimulates release of copious amounts of mucus, and causes contraction of smooth muscle in bronchioles

Fluid pours out of capillaries

Mucus is copiously released

Small respiratory passages (bronchioles) constrict

Variances in Immunity and Inflammation

OBJECTIVES

Cognitive

6.24 Discuss hypersensitivity. (p 146)

6.25 Describe deficiencies in immunity and inflammation. (p 153)

Additional Objectives*

1. Explain the difference between an immediate and a delayed hypersensitivity reaction. (p 146)

2. Describe the four types of hypersensitivity reactions. (p 146–149)

3. List and characterize common autoimmune and isoimmune diseases. (p 150–152)

*These are noncurriculum objectives.

TECHNOLOGY

www.Paramedic.EMSzone.com

- Online Chapter Pretest
- Vocabulary Explorer
- Anatomy Review
- Web Links

Chapter FEATURES

- Case Studies
- Physiology Tips
- Medication Tips
- Paramedic Safety Tips
- Special Needs Tips
- Vital Vocabulary
- Prep Kit

Hypersensitivity

Hypersensitivity is any bodily response to any substance to which a patient has increased sensitivity. This is a generic term for a variety of reactions. Three other terms are used commonly:

1. Allergy – hypersensitivity reaction to the presence of an agent (allergen) that is intrinsically harmless. Examples of common allergens include dog or cat dander, dust, pollen, peanuts, penicillin, codeine, sulfa drugs, shellfish, iodine, and other substances in certain foods.
2. Autoimmunity – production of antibodies or T cells against the tissues of one's own body, producing autoimmune disease or hypersensitivity reactions.
3. Isoimmunity – formation of T cells or antibodies directed against the antigens on another person's cells (typically after the transplantation of an organ or tissues).

The destruction of cells by antibodies or T cells may be either an autoimmune or an isoimmune reaction. A blood transfusion reaction is an example of an isoimmune reaction to another person's red blood cells. When the body forms antibodies against its own tissues, the process is called an autoimmune reaction or response. The disease systemic lupus is an example of an autoimmune response.

Paramedics frequently treat patients who are experiencing different forms of allergic reactions in the field. They also treat patients with medical histories that include many of the conditions introduced in this chapter, such as AIDS, arthritis, lupus, Graves' disease, diabetes, and other diseases that affect patients' immunity.

Mechanisms of Hypersensitivity

A hypersensitivity reaction may be immediate, occurring within seconds to minutes, or delayed, occurring hours to days after exposure to an antigen. The rapidity of symptom evolution depends on the antigen and the type of response the body mounts against it. Hypersensitivity reactions are typically classified into four types: type I, II, III, and IV. The types of hypersensitivity reactions are compared in ▼ Table 9-1.

Type I Hypersensitivity Reactions

A type I hypersensitivity reaction is an immediate, or acute, reaction that occurs in response to a stimulus (eg, bee sting, penicillin, shellfish). The mechanism involves interaction between the stimulus

Table 9-1
Immediate and Delayed Hypersensitivities Compared

	Type I Immediate Hypersensitivity	Type IV Delayed Hypersensitivity

Clinical condition	Hay fever
	Asthma
	Urticaria
	Allergic skin conditions
	Serum sickness
	Anaphylactic shock
		Drug allergies
		Infectious allergies
		   Tuberculosis
		   Rheumatic fever
		   Histoplasmosis
		   Trichinosis
		Contact dermatitis

Onset	Immediate	Delayed
Duration	Short: hours	Prolonged: days or longer

Allergen	Pollen
	Molds
	House dust
	Danders
	Drugs
	Antibiotics
	Soluble proteins and
	   carbohydrates
	Foods
		Drugs
		Antibiotics
		Microorganisms: bacteria, viruses,
		   fungi, animal parasites
		Poison ivy and plant oils
		Plastics and other chemicals
		Fabrics, furs
		Cosmetics

Passive transfer of sensitivity	With serum	With cells or cell fractions of lymphoid series

Adapted from Alcamo, Edward I., *Fundamentals of Microbiology* 6th edition, p. 658, 2001, Jones and Bartlett Publishers.

Medication Tip

An EpiPen is often prescribed to patients who have previously had a serious allergic reaction. These "pens" are carried by patients in their pocketbooks or backpacks and are especially important when patients experience higher risk activities such as camping or hiking. EMS personnel are taught to verify that the medication is actually prescribed for the patient, to ensure it is not out of date, and to recognize the signs and symptoms of anaphylaxis.

Most states have provided treatment protocols that describe how medical direction will authorize the use of an EpiPen by trained EMS providers. They come in two standard sizes: the adult auto-injector, which contains 0.3 mg of medicine, and the pediatric auto-injector, which contains 0.15 mg. These devices are designed to be used in the following manner: (1) Remove the cap. (2) Place the tip against the patient's thigh. (3) Push the auto-injector firmly against the thigh until it activates. (4) Hold the auto-injector in place until the medication is injected. This usually takes about 10 seconds. Be sure to dispose of the EpiPen in a sharps container or the plastic tube in which it is packaged because the needle is exposed and can spread bloodborne pathogens.

alled an antigen, and a preformed antibody of the gE type. **IgE antibodies** work against various antigens and reside on the cell surface of mast cells. When the antibody binds an antigen, the mast cell egranulates, a process that causes the release of istamine (▶ **Figure 9-1**). The released histamine eds back on both mast cells and eosinophils, leading to the release of additional histamine and other mediators. This in turn leads to symptoms. The everity of the symptoms that a particular patient evelops depends on the total extent of mediator elease.

Generally, it is impossible to predict how severe ny given reaction will be. If a person has had a evere reaction in the past, he or she is at an ncreased risk for another one with subsequent ntigen exposures. An IgE-mediated hypersensitivy reaction is also called **anaphylaxis** or an anahylactic reaction. Although some reserve this term or the more severe episodes involving bronchoconriction and cardiovascular collapse, the mechaisms are similar for the entire spectrum of IgE-ediated reactions. You should always assume that ny IgE-mediated reaction could rapidly transition

Case Study

Case Study, Part 1

Your unit is dispatched to a call for difficulty breathing. The address is a familiar one. You know the patient, a 38-year-old man who was diagnosed with acquired immunodeficiency syndrome (AIDS) 2 years ago. Every couple of months or so he requests transport to the local detox center for alcohol abuse. He is a heavy smoker, and it is not clear whether he is compliant with his medication regimen. Today his roommate lets you in and tells you that the patient has been having symptoms of fever, chills, sore throat, and difficulty breathing that has worsened during the last 3 days.

The patient is lying in bed. He appears weak yet is alert to your presence and answers your questions appropriately. He has had a nonproductive cough for 3 days, and today he became extremely short of breath when he tried to get out of bed. His lung sounds are diminished in the right base. His skin is warm and dry. Your partner administers oxygen by nonrebreathing mask, and you obtain his vital signs. He is a high-priority patient due to his respiratory distress.

Initial Assessment

Recording time
0 minutes

Appearance
Weak and mild to moderate distress

Level of consciousness
Alert

Airway
Open

Vital Signs

Pulse rate/quality
112 beats/min, regular and strong

Blood pressure
110/50 mm Hg

Respiratory rate/depth
28 breaths/min, shallow

Question 1: What infectious precautions are needed with this patient?

Question 2: What type of disease is AIDS?

Question 3: Does HIV affect any of the mechanisms of hypersensitivity? If so, how?

CASE STUDY

into a life-threatening event. These reactions need to be treated quickly in the field, and for that reason most out-of-hospital providers are trained in the administration of epinephrine by use of an EpiPen auto-injector (▶ **Figure 9-2**) or by administering a subcutaneous injection as a paramedic might have orders to do.

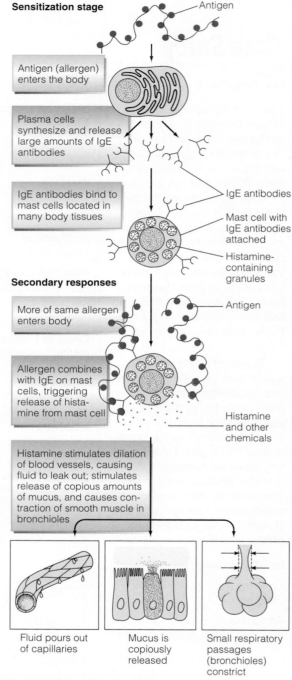

Figure 9-1 Allergic reaction. Antigen stimulates the production of massive amounts of IgE, a type of antibody produced by plasma cells. IgE attaches to mast cells. This is a sensitization stage. When the antigen enters again, it binds to the IgE antibodies on the mast cells, triggering a massive release of histamine and other chemicals. Histamine, in turn, causes blood vessels to dilate and become leaky and promotes increased production of mucus in the respiratory tract. Additionally, mast cell degranulation can also cause bronchospasm in some people.

Paramedic Safety Tip

Latex allergy affects 5% to 10% of health care providers, as well as patients. Many types of medical equipment, in addition to gloves, contain latex rubber or its derivatives (eg, bandages, blood pressure cuffs). Often simply the powder from latex gloves is sufficient to trigger a reaction in a sensitive individual. Reactions follow a typical type I allergic pattern, with symptoms ranging from hives to severe bronchospasm and even cardiac arrest. The treatment is the same as for any other anaphylactic reaction. However, latex reactions are preventable—a variety of latex-free medical supplies are available for EMS providers. At a minimum, ambulances should carry a separate kit with all essential supplies (eg, ECG electrodes, blood pressure cuffs, bandages) in a latex-free version. Failure to have this equipment available may significantly impact your ability to provide proper care to a sick individual who also happens to be allergic to latex.

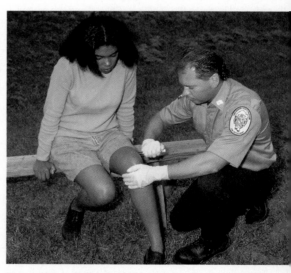

Figure 9-2 An EpiPen auto-injector may be used to administer a preset dose of epinephrine to the patient experiencing a severe allergic reaction.

Other allergic syndromes that also involve Ig but are distinct clinically from anaphylaxis include:

- Allergic rhinitis – an inhaled antigen (eg, pollen) that leads to edema and irritation of the nasal mucosa.
- Bronchial asthma – an inhaled antigen that leads to bronchial constriction, mucus production, and airway inflammation.

- Wheal and flare – a skin-based antigen (eg, insect bite) that leads to localized vasodilation and swelling.
- Food allergy – an ingested antigen (eg, milk) that leads to diarrhea, gastrointestinal distress, and vomiting.

A propensity to type I reactions may be diagnosed through skin tests (eg, patch test, scratch test) and other laboratory procedures (measurement of specific IgE antibody levels). Treatment is avoidance of the antigen. Desensitizing injections may be helpful in severe cases.

Type II Hypersensitivity Reactions

In a type II hypersensitivity reaction, antibodies other than IgE combine with antigens on cells throughout the body. Cells are then destroyed, either by complement or by other antibodies. Type II reactions involve primarily IgG antibodies that attach to a cell surface, react with complement, and cause cell lysis (destruction). This process also destroys many of the body's healthy cells. Histamine release from mast cells is not involved, and IgG-mediated allergic responses occur within a few hours of antigen exposure. Examples of IgG-mediated responses include transfusion reactions and newborn hemolytic disease.

Type III Hypersensitivity Reactions

Type III responses involve primarily IgG antibodies that form immune complexes with antigen to recruit phagocytic cells, such as neutrophils, to a site where they can release inflammatory cytokines. Since histamine release from mast cells is not involved, IgG-mediated allergic responses occur within a few hours of antigen exposure. Reactions may be systemic or localized. The systemic form is called **serum sickness** and results from a large, single exposure to an antigen, such as horse antibody serum. The localized form is called an **Arthus reaction**, which was named for French physiologist Nicholas Maurice Arthus who described the reaction in 1903. Arthus reactions consist of a circumscribed area of vascular inflammation (**vasculitis**). An example of this is farmer's lung, which is a local hypersensitivity reaction in the lung from molds that grow on hay. Arthritis is a common example of an Arthus reaction.

Type IV Hypersensitivity Reactions

Type IV allergic responses are primarily mediated by soluble molecules that are released by specifically activated T cells. These reactions have two subtypes:

Case Study

Case Study, Part 2

You perform a focused physical assessment and obtain a SAMPLE history. The patient's skin is warm and dry. His respiratory effort is slightly labored, especially after he coughs. His SpO$_2$ is 88% and the electrocardiogram shows sinus tachycardia. The presence of a fever together with diminished breath sounds on the right lead you to suspect pneumonia. Patients with AIDS or HIV infection are at great risk for respiratory infections and diseases such as pneumonia and tuberculosis. While you start an IV, your partner administers a bronchodilator nebulizer treatment, which should help the patient breathe easier. The patient complains of headache and increased fatigue in addition to the other symptoms. His roommate brings you the list of his medications and allergies.

Focused Physical Assessment

Recording time
5 minutes

Skin signs
Pale, warm, and dry

Lung sounds
Dry and diminished on the right side
No jugular vein distention or peripheral edema

Vital Signs
Unchanged

Diagnostic Tools

Electrocardiogram
Sinus tachycardia at 112 beats/min

SpO$_2$
88%

Question 4: List the causes of acquired immunodeficiencies.

Question 5: How might a poor diet and nutrition affect immune function and inflammatory response?

CASE STUDY

---

delayed hypersensitivity and cell-mediated cytotoxicity. The first type, **delayed hypersensitivity**, involves lymphocytes and macrophages. T cells respond to an antigen and activate CD4 lymphocytes. These lymphocytes release mediators that are designed to destroy the foreign substance. A well-known example is the reaction to poison ivy. The second type, **cell-mediated cytotoxicity**, involves only sensitized T cells (CD8 lymphocytes or **T killer cells**). These cells kill the antigen-bearing target cells rather than activating the CD4 lymphocyte to do so. The body's response to viral infections is a common example of cell-mediated cytotoxicity. This is also the mechanism by which transplant rejection occurs.

Medication Tip

Many EMS systems have paramedic protocols that incorporate the use of diphenhydramine (Benadryl) for mild to moderate allergic reactions. Benadryl is an antihistamine. It works by suppressing the effects of histamine, a common mediator released during allergic reactions. Benadryl is available over the counter and as a prescription medication in stronger doses. A significant side effect is often drowsiness, leading some physicians to prescribe antihistamines such as centirizine (Zyrtec), which have less of a sedating effect.

Once the cascade of events in anaphylaxis has begun, all of these reactions have the potential to proceed to complete cardiovascular collapse. Epinephrine is the drug of choice for the management of anaphylaxis since there are other mediators involved that need to be blocked as well as histamine. The use of Benadryl by itself (or any other antihistamine) is insufficient and may be dangerous.

Table 9-2
Allergens That Can Cause Hypersensitivity Reactions

Type	Examples
Inhalants	Pollen, dust, smoke, fungi, plastic, odors
Foods	Eggs, milk, wheat, chocolate, strawberries
Drugs	Aspirin, antibiotics, serums, codeine
Infectious agents	Bacteria, viruses, fungi, animal parasites
Contactants	Animals, plants, metals, chemicals
Physical agents	Light, pressure, radiation, heat, cold

Targets of Hypersensitivity

The immune system targets different molecules, depending on the type of hypersensitivity reaction. In allergic reactions, the target is an antigen or **allergen**. Allergens are substances that cause a hypersensitivity reaction, such as those listed in ▲ **Table 9-2**. In autoimmune reactions, the target is a person's own tissues. For reasons that are unclear, normal tolerance of "self" tissues breaks down and the immune system treats the body's own tissues as foreign. In isoimmune diseases, the target is another person's cells (eg, transfusion reaction) or protein (eg, transplant rejection).

Autoimmune and Isoimmune Diseases

Autoimmune reactions may involve humoral or cell-mediated hypersensitivity reactions. Humoral mechanisms involve antibodies against self-antigen (autoantibodies). One of the most important type of autoantibodies is **antinuclear antibodies**. These are antibodies that react with and destroy the nucleus of a cell. The most commonly used clinical test to detect these antibodies examines the microscopic appearance of these antibodies when the cell is treated with a special stain. The stain contains a fluorescent dye that glows green when exposed to ultraviolet light. Various patterns of fluorescence may occur, including speckled (looks like speckles on a speckled jelly bean) and diffuse (the entire nucleus "glows" green). The pattern of nuclear staining suggests the type of antibody that is present in the patient's serum, which can help to identify the type of autoimmune disease an individual has. Common autoimmune and isoimmune diseases include the following:

- **Graves' disease** – an autoimmune disease caused by thyroid-stimulating immunoglobulins or thyroid-growth immunoglobulins. These antibodies activate receptors for thyroid-stimulating hormone (TSH), causing increased activity by the thyroid gland. In addition to hyperthyroidism, Graves' disease is associated with characteristic changes in the eyes and the skin. The eye changes consist of lid retraction, stare, and **exophthalmus** (protrusion of the eyes). The skin changes (pretibial myxedema) consist of localized edematous skin in the pretibial area.

- Diabetes mellitus – Type 1 diabetes mellitus is now considered an autoimmune disease. Although the initial instigating insult is unknown, some agent stimulates the body to produce autoantibodies against beta cells in the pancreas that produce insulin. The result is a deficiency of insulin and diabetes. Many researchers hypothesize that the initial event is some type of a viral infection.

- **Rheumatoid arthritis** – a chronic systemic disease that affects the entire body and is one of the most common forms of arthritis. It is characterized by inflammation of the **synovium** (the connective tissue membrane lining

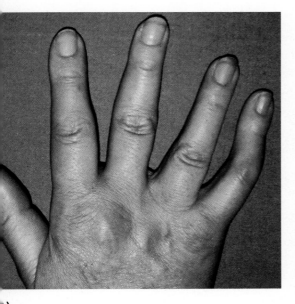

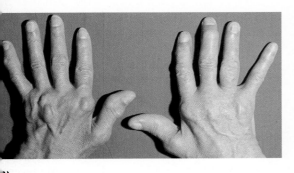

gure 9-3 Rheumatoid arthritis. **A.** Early examples of swelling
f the knuckle joints as a result of inflammation. **B.** More
dvanced changes, illustrating joint deformities and ulnar
eviation of fingers.

Case Study

Case Study, Part 3

By the time you have finished starting the IV, the oxygen and bronchodilator appear to have improved the patient's respiratory effort. The patient is ready to be moved to the ambulance. Because your patient may have had a severe reaction, the administration of a corticosteroid such as methylpred-nisolone (Solu-Medrol) might be effective in reducing hypoxemia and the need for intubation. You contact medical control en route to discuss this option. Before you call, you reassess the patient's condition and take another set of vital signs.

Ongoing Assessment

Recording time
20 minutes

Appearance and mental status
The patient appears more alert at this time.

Vital Signs

Pulse rate/quality
108 beats/min, regular and strong

Blood pressure
114/54 mm Hg

Respiratory rate/depth
24 breaths/min and regular

Diagnostic Tools

Electrocardiogram
Sinus tachycardia at 108 beats/min

SpO_2
96%

Question 6: Immune thrombocytopenia purpura (ITP) is a common disorder in patients in the asymptomatic stage of HIV infection. What is purpura?

Question 7: Since immunodeficiency disorders are relatively uncommon, when should they be considered?

CASE STUDY

the joint) with resulting pain, stiffness, warmth, redness, and swelling. Inflammatory cells release enzymes that cause damage to bone and cartilage. The involved joint can lose its shape and alignment, resulting in pain and loss of movement, as illustrated in ▲ **Figure 9-3**. Rheumatoid arthritis is associated with the formation of **rheumatoid factor**, IgM antibodies to tissue IgG. In the joints, the synovial membrane is thickened due to infiltration of inflammatory cells (lymphocytes).

- **Myasthenia gravis** – an acquired auto-immune disease that is characterized by autoimmune attack on the nerve-muscle junction. The circulating autoantibodies cause abnormal muscle fatigability and typically involve the smallest motor units first, such as

the extraocular muscles. This produces *ptosis* (droopy eyelid) and *diplopia* (double vision). Other muscles may be involved, causing problems with swallowing (*dysphagia*). Characteristically, repeated contraction of the affected muscles makes the symptoms worse. The symptoms are promptly reversed with the medication edrophonium (Tensilon), a short-acting anticholinesterase. Two thirds of patients with myasthenia gravis have thymic abnormalities, the most common being thymic hyperplasia. A minority of patients have a tumor of the thymus, called a **thymoma**.

- **Immune thrombocytopenia purpura** – a blood disorder. The patient forms antibodies to blood platelets that cause their destruction. Thrombocytopenia describes a decrease in blood platelets. Purpura are purplish areas of the skin and mucous membranes (such as the lining of the mouth) where bleeding has occurred as a result of decreased or ineffective platelets. Some cases of ITP are caused by drugs, and others are associated with infection, pregnancy, or immune disorders such as systemic lupus erythematosus. About half of all cases are classified as "idiopathic," meaning the cause is unknown.

Bleeding is the main symptom of ITP and can include bruising and tiny red dots on the skin or mucous membranes. In some instances bleeding from the nose, gums, and digestive or urinary tracts may also occur. Rarely, bleeding within the brain occurs.

Treatment of idiopathic ITP is based on the severity of the symptoms and the patient's platelet count. In some cases, no therapy is needed. In most cases, drugs that alter the immune system's attack on the platelets are prescribed. These include corticosteroids (eg, prednisone) and/or IV infusions of immunoglobulin. Another treatment that usually results in an increased number of platelets is removal of the spleen, the organ that destroys antibody-coated platelets.

- **Isoimmune neonatal neutropenia** – Isoimmune neonatal neutropenia occurs when anti-neutrophil antibodies from the mother cross via the placenta and cause neutropenia that lasts 2 to 4 weeks. **Neutropenia** is a decreased number of circulating neutrophils. This disease is seen only rarely.

- **Systemic lupus erythematosus (SLE)** – a chronic disease with many manifestations. SLE is an autoimmune disease in which the body's own immune system is directed against the body's own tissues. The etiology of SLE is not known. Although this disease is more common in young women, it can occur in either sex at any age. The production of autoantibodies leads to immune complex formation. Immune complex deposition in many tissues leads to the manifestations of the disease (▼ **Figure 9-4**). Immune complexes can be deposited in glomeruli, skin, lungs, synovium, mesothelium, and other places. Many SLE patients develop renal complications.

Symptoms include arthritis, a red rash over the nose and cheeks, fatigue, weakness, fever, and photosensitivity. Glomerulonephritis (kidney disease), pericarditis, anemia, and neuritis may develop.

- Rh and ABO isoimmunization – **Rh factor** is an antigen present in the erythrocytes (red blood cells) of about 85% of people. Persons having the factor are designated Rh-positive; those lacking the factor, Rh-negative. Blood for transfusions must be classified for Rh factor, as well as for ABO blood group, to prevent possible incompatibility reactions. If an Rh-negative person receives Rh-positive blood, hemolysis and anemia can result. A similar reaction can occur if an Rh-negative mother exposes an Rh-positive fetus to antibodies to

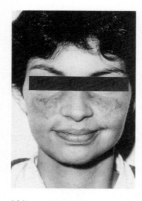
(A)

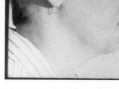
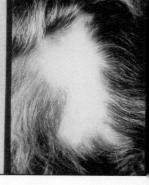
(B)

Figure 9-4 Systemic lupus erythematosus. Two patients showing some of the symptoms of systemic lupus erythematosus (SLE). **A.** The butterfly rash on the face. Note how the rash extends out to the cheeks like the wings of a butterfly. **B.** A young girl displaying the loss of hair that accompanies some cases of SLE.

the factor. This hemolytic disease of the new-born is illustrated in ▼ Figure 9-5.

Immune and Inflammation Deficiencies

Immunodeficiency is an abnormal condition in which some part of the body's immune system is inadequate, and consequently resistance to infectious disease is decreased. Immunodeficiency may be congenital or acquired. Diseases involving congenital immunodeficiency include:

- **Severe combined immunodeficiency disease (SCID)** – Patients with this disease have defects that involve lymphoid stem cells, and therefore both T cells (cellular immunity) and B cells (humoral immunity) are affected. Patients are at risk for infection with all types of organisms (eg, bacteria, mycobacteria, fungi, viruses, and parasites). There are two forms of this disease and both are inherited.

- **X-linked agammaglobulinemia of Bruton** – This is one of the most common forms of primary immunodeficiency. This disease, which is found in male infants, is caused by a defect in the differentiation of pre-B cells to B cells. The result is markedly decreased levels of all immunoglobulins and of mature B lymphocytes. T lymphocytes function normally. Therefore, patients develop recurrent pyrogenic infections but have no problems with fungal and viral infections because cell-

mediated immunity is unaffected. These infections begin in affected infants at about 6 months of age when maternal immunoglobulin levels have decreased.

- **Isolated deficiency of IgA** – Probably the most common form of immunodeficiency, this disease results from a block in the terminal

Case Study

Case Study, Part 4

Completion of Case Study

En route to the hospital the patient received IV Solu-Medrol and continued nebulizer treatments. His respiratory effort continued to improve during transport. The emergency department staff recognized the patient immediately. Later on that day as you are delivering another patient to the ED, you learn that the patient did have pneumonia, a type called *Pneumocystis carinii.*

Pneumocystis carinii pneumonia is caused by a fungus that is common in patients with depressed cell-mediated immunity. More than 80% of patients with AIDS have this infection at some time if prophylaxis is not given. Patients with HIV infection become susceptible to *Pneumocystic carinii* pneumonia when their CD4 cell counts are low.

Signs and symptoms include fever, dyspnea, and dry, nonproductive cough that develops acutely over days or subacutely over weeks. Other symptoms include headache, fatigue, sore throat, vomiting, chills, and diarrhea.

CASE STUDY

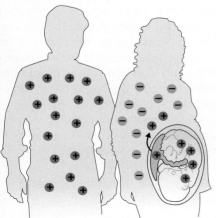

(A) Hemolytic disease of the newborn can develop when an Rh-positive man and an Rh-negative woman have a baby.

(B) When an Rh-negative woman gives birth to an Rh-positive baby, Rh antigens from the child's blood enter the woman's blood.

(C) The antigens stimulate her immune system to produce Rh antibodies that circulate in her blood, but since the baby has already been born, there is no effect on the child.

(D) In a future pregnancy, if the baby is Rh-positive, the Rh antibodies will cross the placenta and enter the baby's blood.

(E) The Rh antibodies attack the baby's red blood cells by uniting with Rh antigens on their surface; they damage the cells, leading to severe anemia and hemolytic disease.

Figure 9-5 Hemolytic disease of the newborn.

differentiation of B lymphocytes. Most patients are asymptomatic, but some may develop chronic sinus infections. Patients also have an increased incidence of autoimmune disease.

Causes of acquired immunodeficiencies include:

- Nutritional deficiencies – Any nutritional deficiency can hamper normal immune function and the inflammatory response. Nutritional deficiencies have been shown to result in depression of bone marrow function and reduction in white blood cell development. A lack of protein in the diet decreases the ability of the liver to manufacture inflammatory mediators and plasma proteins.
- Trauma-related deficiencies – It is believed that the stress of trauma can cause immunodeficiency. Other contributors to this condition can include hypoperfusion or shock, mediator production, damage to vital organs, and the decreased nutrition occurring during trauma states.
- Iatrogenic (treatment-induced) deficiencies – Iatrogenic immunodeficiency is most frequently caused by drugs. Corticosteroids, taken orally or inhaled, suppress the immune system. Often, this results in therapeutic benefit to the patient. In a small number of patients, however, the resulting immunosuppression leads to other diseases (eg, tuberculosis). Usually physicians are very careful about the prescribed duration of therapy because of the potential adverse effects. Idiosyncratic reactions to antibiotics may result in bone marrow suppression, as is the case with chemotherapeutic drugs for cancer. Many cases of bone marrow suppression in cancer are direct and predictable side effects of chemotherapy, and not true idiosyncratic, "out of the blue," reactions.
- Stress-related deficiencies – Physical or mental stress has been shown to result in a decrease in the white blood cell and lymphocyte function, as well as a decreased production of various antibodies.
- <u>**Acquired immunodeficiency syndrome (AIDS)**</u> – an immunodeficiency disease that is caused by the RNA retrovirus HIV (human

Table 9-3

Sequence of Events in HIV Infections and Their Significance

Event	Significance
HIV invades CD4+ cells and becomes part of cell DNA	Individual is infected for life
Virus proliferates in infected cells and sheds virus particles	Virus present in blood and body fluids
Body forms anti-HIV antibody	Antibody is a marker of infection but is not protective
Progressive destruction of helper T cells, with relative excess of suppressor T cells	Compromised cell-mediated immunity
Immune defenses collapse	Opportunistic infections Neoplasms

Adapted from Crowley, Leonard, *An Introduction to Human Disease Pathology and Pathophysiology Correlations* 6th edition, Table 8-2, p. 163, 2004, Jones and Bartlett.

immunodeficiency virus). HIV binds to the CD4 surface protein of helper T lymphocytes, infects these cells, and kills them. This causes decreased humoral and cell-mediated reactions. The sequence of events in HIV infections and their significance are described in ▲ Table 9-3.

Replacement therapy is available for some types of immunodeficiencies (eg, common variable immunodeficiency). Intravenous gamma globulin has been used in the therapy of a number of immunologic disorders of the nervous system, especially myasthenia gravis and inflammatory neuropathies, with considerable success. Bone marrow transplantation may restore immune competence in persons with acquired causes of immunodeficiency, such as following chemotherapy for cancer. In the future, gene therapy may be useful for treatment of both congenital and acquired causes of immunodeficiency. Currently gene therapy is purely experimental and not clinically available for use.

Several disorders result from acquired or inherited defects in leukocyte function. As a result, the inflammatory response may be defective.

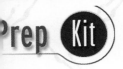

Chapter Summary

Hypersensitivity is an increased bodily response to any substance to which a patient is abnormally sensitive. This is a generic term for a variety of reactions. Three other terms are used commonly: allergy, autoimmunity, and isoimmunity.

A hypersensitivity reaction may be immediate, occurring within seconds to minutes, or delayed, occurring hours to days after exposure to the antigen.

- There are four types of hypersensitivity reactions. Type I reactions involve an interaction between an antigen and an IgE antibody. Type II reactions involve primarily IgG antibodies that attach to a cell surface, react with complement, and cause cell lysis. Type III responses involve primarily IgG antibodies that form immune complexes with antigen and complement to recruit phagocytic cells, such as neutrophils, to a site where they can release inflammatory cytokines. Type IV allergic responses are primarily

mediated by soluble molecules that are released by specifically activated T cells.

- The immune system targets different molecules, depending on the type of hypersensitivity reaction. Autoimmune reactions may involve humoral or cell-mediated hypersensitivity reactions. Types of autoimmune or isoimmune diseases include Graves' disease, rheumatoid arthritis, myasthenia gravis, ITP, isoimmune neonatal neutropenia, SLE, and Rh and ABO isoimmunization.

- Immunodeficiency may be congenital or acquired. Diseases involving congenital immunodeficiency include SCID, X-linked agammaglobulinemia of Bruton, and isolated deficiency of IgA. Acquired causes include nutritional deficiencies, iatrogenic deficiencies, trauma, stress, and AIDS. Several disorders result from acquired or inherited defects in leukocyte function. As a result, the inflammatory response may be defective.

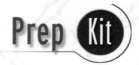

Vital Vocabulary

acquired immunodeficiency syndrome (AIDS) An immunodeficiency disease caused by the RNA retrovirus HIV (human immunodeficiency virus).

allergen Any substance that causes a hypersensitivity reaction.

allergy Hypersensitivity reaction to the presence of an agent (allergen) that is intrinsically harmless.

anaphylaxis A severe hypersensitivity reaction that, in its worst case, involves bronchoconstriction and cardiovascular collapse.

antinuclear antibodies One of the most important types of autoantibodies that react with and destroy the nucleus of a cell.

Arthus reaction A local reaction involving vascular inflammation in response to an IgG-mediated allergic response.

autoimmunity The production of antibodies or T cells against the tissues of a person's own body, producing autoimmune disease or a hypersensitivity reaction.

cell-mediated cytotoxicity A type IV allergic reaction that only involves sensitized T cells.

delayed hypersensitivity A type IV allergic reaction involving lymphocytes and macrophages.

exophthalmus Protrusion of the eyes.

Graves' disease An autoimmune disease caused by thyroid-stimulating immunoglobulins or thyroid-growth immunoglobulins.

hypersensitivity A generic term for bodily responses to a substance to which a patient is abnormally sensitive.

IgE antibodies Antibodies to various antigens that reside on the cell surface of mast cells.

immune thrombocytopenia purpura (ITP) A blood disorder in which the patient forms antibodies to blood platelets that cause their destruction.

immunodeficiency An abnormal condition in which some part of the body's immune system is inadequate, and consequently resistance to infectious disease is decreased.

isoimmune neonatal neutropenia Neutropenia that occurs when antineutrophil antibodies from the mother cross via the placenta.

isoimmunity Formation of antibodies or T cells that are directed against antigens or another person's cells.

isolated deficiency of IgA A form of immunodeficiency that results from a block in the terminal differentiation of B lymphocytes.

myasthenia gravis An acquired autoimmune disease that is characterized by circulating antibodies to the acetylcholine receptors at the myoneural junction; antibodies cause abnormal muscle fatigability.

neutropenia A condition involving a decreased number of circulating neutrophils.

rheumatoid arthritis A chronic systemic disease that affects the entire body and is one of the most common forms of arthritis.

rheumatoid factor IgM antibodies to tissue IgG.

Rh factor An antigen present in the erythrocytes (red blood cells) of about 85% of people.

serum sickness An IgG-mediated allergic reaction that results from a large single exposure to an antigen (see Arthus reaction).

severe combined immunodeficiency disease (SCID) A disease caused by defects in lymphoid stem cells associated with insufficiency in both both T cells (cellular immunity) and B cells (humoral immunity).

synovium The connective tissue lining of the joints.

systemic lupus erythematosus (SLE) A chronic autoimmune disease in which the body's own immune system is directed against the body's own tissues.

thymoma A tumor of the thymus.

T killer cells Cells released during a type IV allergic reaction that kill antigen-bearing target cells.

vasculitis An inflammation of the blood vessels.

X-linked agammaglobulinemia of Bruton A primary immunodeficiency in male infants caused by a defect in the differentiation of pre-B cells to B cells.

Case Study Answers

Question 1: What infectious precautions are needed with this patient?

Answer: The patient is presenting with respiratory distress and fever; therefore an oxygen mask should be placed on the patient and a mask will be appropriate for the EMT-P to decrease the risk of transmission of the infection. AIDS and HIV are transmitted by the bloodborne mechanism. They are also spread by sexual transmission. It is appropriate to wear disposable gloves and an eyeshield when suctioning, or if there is any possibility that blood may splatter.

Question 2: What type of disease is AIDS?

Answer: AIDS is an immunodeficiency disease that is caused by an RNA retrovirus called HIV (human immunodeficiency virus).

Question 3: Does HIV affect any of the mechanisms of hypersensitivity? If so, how?

Answer: HIV infection results in a loss of normal CD4 helper T lymphocytes. This leads to a decreased ability of the body to mount a type IV delayed hypersensitivity reaction, which makes the patient more susceptible to viral, fungal, and tuberculous infections.

Question 4: List the causes of acquired immunodeficiencies.

Answer: Causes of acquired immunodeficiencies include poor nutrition, iatrogenic causes, traumatic injury, mental or physical stress, and AIDS or HIV infection.

Question 5: How might a poor diet and nutrition affect immune function and inflammatory response?

Answer: Any nutritional deficiency can hinder normal immune function and the inflammatory response. Poor nutrition results in decreased production of white blood cells, inflammatory mediators, and plasma proteins.

Question 6: Immune thrombocytopenia purpura (ITP) is a common disorder in patients in the asymptomatic stage of HIV infection. What is purpura?

Answer: Purpura refers to purplish areas of the skin and mucous membrane such as the lining of the mouth.

Question 7: Since immunodeficiency disorders are relatively uncommon, when should they be considered?

Answer: Patients with frequent infections, severe infections, or infections that are resistant to treatment may have underlying immunodeficiency disorders.

CASE STUDY ANSWERS

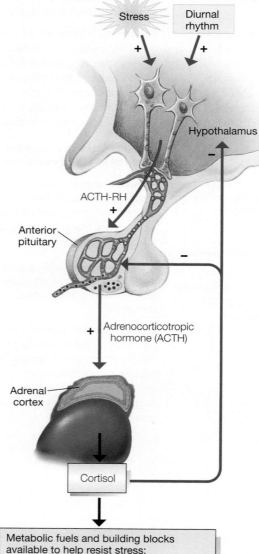

Stress

Diurnal
rhythm

+ +

Hypothalamus

−

ACTH-RH

+

Anterior
pituitary

−

+ Adrenocorticotropic
hormone (ACTH)

Adrenal
cortex

Cortisol

Metabolic fuels and building blocks
available to help resist stress:

• Increases blood concentration of
  glucose (by stimulating gluconeogenesis and inhibiting glucose uptake)
• Increases blood concentration of
  amino acids (by stimulating protein
  degradation)
• Increases blood concentration of fatty
  acids (by stimulating the breakdown of fat)

OBJECTIVES

Cognitive

6.29 Describe neuroendocrine regulation. (p 160)

6.30 Discuss the inter-relationships between stress, coping, and illness. (p 164–168)

Additional Objectives*

1. Discuss the concept of stress and its triad of manifestations in the body. (p 160)

2. Describe the general adaptation syndrome. (p 160–161)

3. Describe the function of the life-change unit and the Hassles Scale. (p 162–163)

4. List ways a paramedic can lead a less stressful life and maintain better overall health. (p 167–168)

*These are noncurriculum objectives.

www.Paramedic.EMSzone.com

TECHNOLOGY

- Online Chapter Pretest
- Vocabulary Explorer
- Anatomy Review
- Web Links

Chapter FEATURES

- Case Studies
- Physiology Tips
- Medication Tips
- Paramedic Safety Tips
- Special Needs Tips
- Vital Vocabulary
- Prep Kit

Concept of Stress

Stress is the medical term for a wide range of strong external stimuli, both physiological and psychological, which can cause a physiological response called the general adaptation syndrome. Usually, the response to stress is appropriate and beneficial. However, an unchecked stress response can result in numerous deleterious outcomes, including:

- Chemical dependency
- Heart attack
- Stroke
- Depression
- Headache
- Abdominal pain

The **general adaptation syndrome**, a term described by Hans Selye in the 1920s, characterizes a three-stage reaction to stressors, both physical (eg, injury) and emotional (eg, loss of a loved one).

Stage 1: Alarm Reaction

The first stage of the general adaptation syndrome is termed the **alarm reaction**. Catecholamine release, described below, leads to the "fight-or-flight"

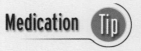

Medication Tip

A number of the medications carried by the paramedic involve the actions of adrenergic receptor sites. Adrenergic receptors respond to the neurotransmitters epinephrine and norepinephrine acting on the sympathetic response. Drugs that mimic the functions of the sympathetic nervous system are called sympathomimetic drugs. Examples of these drugs used in the out-of-hospital setting are dobutamine, dopamine, and epinephrine.

response. Normally, this response prepares the body to deal with stress, but it can also weaken the immune system, leading to infection.

The body reacts to stress first by releasing **catecholamines**, chemical compounds derived from the amino acid tyrosine that act as hormones or neurotransmitters. Catecholamines are soluble, so they circulate dissolved in blood. The most abundant catecholamines are epinephrine (adrenaline), norepinephrine (noradrenaline), and dopamine. They are produced mainly from the

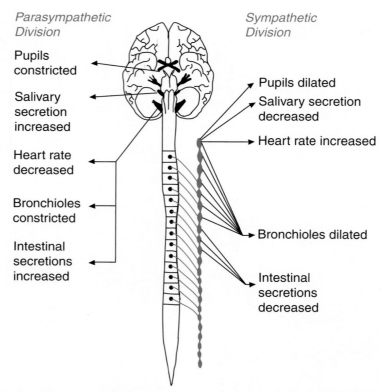

Parasympathetic Division

Pupils constricted

Salivary secretion increased

Heart rate decreased

Bronchioles constricted

Intestinal secretions increased

Sympathetic Division

Pupils dilated

Salivary secretion decreased

Heart rate increased

Bronchioles dilated

Intestinal secretions decreased

Figure 10-1 The sympathetic and parasympathetic systems. Internal organs are typically innervated by neural fibers from both sympathetic and parasympathetic divisions.

Physiology (Tip)

Physiologist Walter Cannon is credited with coining the phrase "fight-or-flight" in his description of how the human body deals with acute stress. Cannon closely studied the stress reaction and how the body prepares to attack aggressors or to adequately fuel the body so that it is able to flee from predators. Cannon described four stages of the fight-or-flight response:

- **Stage One** – Stimuli from one or more of the body's senses are sent to the brain.
- **Stage Two** – After the brain decides if the stimulus is a threat or a nonthreat, it will either end the response for a nonthreatening stimulus or activate the nervous and endocrine systems to prepare for the body's initial response or escape.
- **Stage Three** – The body is in a "ready state" or heightened awareness or arousal waiting for the threat to pass.
- **Stage Four** – The body returns to the normal state of homeostasis once the threat is gone. Homeostasis may be thought of as a "dynamic steady state." Various systems in the body are in balance, but the body is ready to "jump into action" if warranted.

adrenal medulla and the postganglionic fibers of the sympathetic nervous system. The role of the sympathetic and parasympathetic nervous systems is illustrated in ◄ **Figure 10-1**. Adrenaline acts as a neurotransmitter in the central nervous system and as a hormone in the blood. Noradrenaline is primarily a neurotransmitter of the peripheral sympathetic nervous system but is also present in the blood (mostly through "spillover" from the synapses of the sympathetic system).

Stage 2: Resistance Stage

Stage 2, the <u>resistance stage</u>, is the body's way of adapting to stressors. It does this primarily by stimulating the adrenal gland to secrete corticosteroid hormones that increase the blood glucose level and maintain blood pressure:

- Glucocorticoids – The most significant glucocorticoid in the body is cortisol. It controls carbohydrate, fat, and protein metabolism. Cortisol also has potent anti-inflammatory actions.
- Mineralocorticoids – Predominantly aldosterone; mineralocorticoids control electrolyte

Case Study

Case Study, Part 1

Your unit has been dispatched for a suicide attempt. Police are on the scene talking with the patient, and they advise you that it is safe to enter. The patient had taken a garden hose and some duct tape and used it to pump exhaust from his muffler into his vehicle compartment in an attempt to take his life. As you approach the patient you observe that he is alert, crying, and seems to be refusing to cooperate with the police. There is an older couple talking with one of the officers. Apparently his grandparents found him in the vehicle that was parked on their front lawn. They said he had been drinking last night and was distressed over the recent break-up with his girlfriend.

While you listen to the patient bargaining with the officer you consider his affect, behavior, body language, tone of speech, stress level, and the possibility of him becoming physically combative. You remember from your EMT-Basic training that "all suicidal patients are potentially homicidal," so you are caring yet very cautious with the patient. You can see that his respiratory effort is good and he has no trouble speaking. His skin color appears normal. At this point he is not ready to be touched, but the police have given him no choice. He will be going to the hospital in your ambulance.

Initial Assessment

Recording time
0 minutes

Appearance
Distraught

Level of consciousness
Alert

Airway
Open

Vital Signs

Respiratory rate/depth
18 breaths/min, good effort

Skin signs
Skin color is a normal tone.

Question 1: What is stress?

Question 2: What is general adaptation syndrome and what are its three stages?

Question 3: What is the role of cortisol in a stress response?

CASE STUDY

and water levels in the body, mainly by promoting sodium retention by the kidney.

Continuation of stress and accompanying corticosteroid release eventually leads to fatigue, lapses in concentration, irritability, and lethargy.

Stage 3: Exhaustion Stage

After a long period of stress, the person enters the <u>exhaustion stage</u>. The adrenal glands become depleted, leading to decreased blood glucose levels.

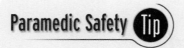

During the past three decades there have been a number of studies on the psychological stress levels in paramedics. The studies that seek to evaluate stress levels and compare them usually examine life-change units, or LCUs. These LCUs were originally described in the Life Chart Theory by Adolph Meyer and further explored by researchers Thomas Holmes and Richard Rahe in their article in the *Journal of Psychosomatic Research*. The researchers used the "Social Readjustment Rating Scale" that ranks 43 stress-producing events in a person's life and provides a weighed score for each event according to the stress potential and degree of disruption and readjustment necessary to deal with the event. The scale, shown in ▼ **Table 10-1**, describes a score of 150 or lower as the normal range of stress. A score between 200 and 299 would be considered a moderate life crisis, and over 300 would indicate a major life crisis. The authors predicted that a score above 150 LCU could be associated with disease and illness (eg, heart attacks). In a study done with the Houston Fire Department paramedics in the late 1970s, it was found that the average score was 124 LCUs. The

Table 10-1
Social Readjustment Rating Scale

Rank	Life Event	LCU	Rank	Life Event	LCU
1	Death of a spouse	100	23	Son or daughter leaving home	29
2	Divorce	73	24	Trouble with in-laws	29
3	Marital separation	65	25	Outstanding personal achievement	28
4	Jail term	63	26	Spouse begins or stops work	26
5	Death of close family member	63	27	Begin or end school	26
6	Personal injury or illness	53	28	Change in living conditions	25
7	Marriage	50	29	Revision of personal habits	24
8	Fired at work	47	30	Trouble with boss	23
9	Marital reconciliation	45	31	Change in work hours or conditions	20
10	Retirement	45	32	Change in residence	20
11	Change in health of family member	44	33	Change in schools	20
12	Pregnancy	40	34	Change in recreation	19
13	Sexual dysfunction	39	35	Change in church activities	19
14	Gain of new family member	39	36	Change in social activities	18
15	Business readjustment	39	37	Mortgage or loan less than $10,000	17
16	Change in financial status	38	38	Change in sleeping habits	16
17	Death of close friend	37	39	Change in number of family get-togethers	15
18	Change to different line of work	36	40	Change in eating habits	13
19	Change in number of arguments with spouse	35	41	Vacation	13
20	Mortgage over $100,000	31	42	Christmas	12
21	Foreclosure of mortgage or loan	30	43	Minor violation of the law	11
22	Change in responsibilities at work	29			

Check off those events that currently apply to your life and add up the corresponding points or Life-Change Units. A score below 150 is thought to be within the range of normal stress. A score between 150 and 199 suggests a mild life crisis; between 200 and 299 points suggests a moderate life crisis; above 300 points is indicative of a major life crisis. (Reprinted by permission of the publisher from "The Social Readjustment Rating Scale" by T.H. Holmes and R. Rahe, Journal of Psychosomatic Research, vol. 11, pp. 213-218. Copyright 1967 by Elsevier Science Inc.)

Paramedic Safety Tip

same study was repeated in 1979 with the New York City paramedics, and the average score was 335 LCUs.

More recent research by Richard Lazarus has investigated the accumulation of daily stressors, utilizing the so-called Hassles Scale (▼ Table 10-2). Lazarus defined these "hassles" as daily interactions with the environment that were essentially negative. He found the hassles to be based on unmet expectations that trigger an anger response. He hypothesized that we all need a balance of emotional experiences that are both positive (highs) and negative (lows). The people who do not have exposure to life's "highs" are susceptible to disease and illness. This theory has been well received, although some researchers argue that perception plays an even more important role in the impact of stressors. It is clear that regardless of the theory, all stressors are directly connected to the well-being of the person.

Table 10-2
The Measurement of Hassles

Recently psychologists have examined the role of minor stressors in the development of disease and illness. The following sample items from the Hassles Scale (Kanner et al.) indicate what might be perceived to be everyday hassles or petty annoyances.

1 = somewhat severe; 2 = moderately severe; 3 = extremely severe

Directions: Hassles are small irritants that can range from minor annoyances to fairly major pressures, problems, or difficulties. They can occur few or many times. Listed below are a number of ways in which a person can feel hassled. First, circle the hassles that have happened to you in the past month. Then look at the numbers to the right of the items you circled. Indicate by circling a 1, 2, or 3 how severe each of these circled hassles has been for you in the past month. If a hassle did not occur in the last month, do not circle it.

1. Not getting enough sleep	1	2	3
2. Job dissatisfaction	1	2	3
3. Use of alcohol	1	2	3
4. Inconsiderate smokers	1	2	3
5. Thoughts about death	1	2	3
6. Health of family	1	2	3
7. Not enough money for clothing	1	2	3
8. Concerns about owing money	1	2	3
9. Fear of rejection	1	2	3
10. Concern about weight	1	2	3

The Hassles Scale has over 118 items. These questions provide only a sample and thus it is not possible to evaluate your personal daily hassles from this set. The second part of this scale is referred to as the Uplift Scale, a series of 136 questions to determine what events promote joy and happiness. The following is a sample.

1. Being with younger people	1	2	3
2. Entertainment	1	2	3
3. Laughing	1	2	3
4. Being one with the world	1	2	3
5. Hugging or kissing	1	2	3

Reproduced with permission from Taylor, S., *Health Psychology*, pp. 10, 221, 1998, McGraw-Hill, New York.

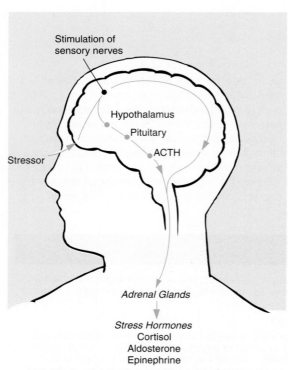

Figure 10-2 The corticotropin axis. The stress response includes increased neural excitability, increased cardiovascular activity (heart rate, stroke volume, cardiac output, blood pressure), increased metabolic activity (gluconeogenesis, protein mobilization, fat mobilization), increased sodium retention, increase in neurological sweating, change in salivation, and change in GI system tonus and motility.

The result is decreased stress tolerance, progressive mental and physical exhaustion, illness, and collapse. At this point, the body's immune system is compromised, reducing a person's ability to resist disease significantly. Heart attack, high blood pressure, or severe infection may result.

The hypothalamic-pituitary-adrenal axis (HPA axis) is a major part of the neuroendocrine system that controls reactions to stress. The HPA axis triggers a set of interactions among glands, hormones, and parts of the mid-brain that mediate the general adaptation syndrome. Continued stress, however, leads to loss of normal control mechanisms. As a result, the adrenals continue to produce cortisol, which exhausts the stress mechanism and leads to fatigue and depression. Cortisol also interferes with serotonin activity, furthering the depressive effect. The impact of the HPA axis is illustrated in ▲ Figure 10-2.

The leading causes of death in adults are dominated by lifestyle diseases, such as heart attacks and strokes, chronic lung diseases, and diabetes. Lifestyle diseases are those whose pathology develops over years and are often preventable through the alteration of habits and behavioral changes during a person's younger years. The lifestyle of a paramedic in a busy EMS system can be very stressful and action-filled. Often the behaviors of paramedics, such as unhealthy eating practices and a lack of overall fitness, can set them up for the inability to properly cope with stress in the field.

Consistently high cortisol levels lead to suppression of the immune system through increased production of interleukin-6, an immune system messenger. This coincides with research findings indicating that stress and depression have a negative effect on the immune system. Reduced immunity makes the body more susceptible to everything from colds and flu to cancer. For example, the incidence of serious illness, including cancer, is significantly higher among people who have suffered the death of a spouse in the previous year.

People experiencing severe, prolonged stress may contract diseases as a result of immune deficiency and may even die of these diseases. Although the stress does not cause the death directly, it does cause the body to lose its ability to fight disease in its effort to manage the stress. The immune deficiency brought on by chronic stress leads to life-threatening conditions such as serious infections or cancer. For this reason, it is very important that we recognize the cause of stresses and, as far as possible, eliminate those causes to maintain good health.

Stress causes the body to release fat and cholesterol into the bloodstream, which in turn leads to clogging of the arteries. This may result in a heart attack or stroke. Many people start drinking alcohol to excess to combat their stress. Other manifestations of chronic stress include depression, headaches, insomnia, ulcers, and asthma.

Fortunately, this immune suppression process can be corrected with psychotherapy, medication, or any number of other positive influences that restore hope and a feeling of self-esteem. The ability of human beings to recover from adversity is remarkable.

Essential Health of the Paramedic

According to the World Health Organization, health is not merely the absence of disease or infirmity. It is a state of complete physical, mental, and social well-being. Health is the vital principle that enables us to meet and overcome the challenges of the day. For this to occur, preventive measures, medicine, and surgery are not enough. We must enlist all our functions, along with the body, mind, and spirit, to attain true health.

Being physically fit involves many components, including aerobic conditioning (cardiovascular fitness), strength, speed, endurance, flexibility, balance, coordination, body composition, and mental attitude. If you do not already have a fitness plan, it's time to start one. Do not compare yourself with others when you are defining your fitness goals. For help in developing your personal fitness goals, you can consult with your physician, talk to an athletic trainer, or review materials available from the President's Counsel of Fitness. Expect it to take a minimum of 6 to 12 weeks to see the effects of training and have fun during the process (▶ Figure 10-3). Make your goals realistic and attainable so you will stick with the regimen you've chosen.

A baseline and ongoing physical exam is an essential part of the paramedic's well-being and a good place to start. It is useful to keep documentation of your health in case you become sick or injured. Avoiding personal injury should be a high priority. Paramedics, as part of their routine patient care, have to be able to lift and move patients of all sizes. This places paramedics at an increased risk for back injuries, so being personally fit can go a long way in preventing them. Proper lifting techniques along with good physical conditioning will greatly reduce the incidence of back injury. Attention should be given to strengthening the abdominal and leg muscles because these are the primary muscles used when lifting patients.

Think seriously about improving your endurance as well. When responding to a call for difficulty breathing that requires you to climb several flights of stairs, you should not be more short of breath than the patient! Routine aerobic exercise lasting at least 20 minutes, three times a week, begins to improve your cardiac stroke volume and increase your physical endurance.

To maintain intelligence, you must continually retrain the brain; just as vision fades, the human brain also deteriorates with age. Our ability to recognize numbers in a test sequence starts to decline after the age of 25. Stimulating the central nervous system with physical activity may delay the loss of nerve cells in the brain by increasing the level of oxygen in the brain. This would suggest that exercise may become more important to brainpower as we age. If so, the saying "Use it or lose it" applies as much to the brain as it does to the muscles.

The Importance of Diet and Nutrition

The Standard American Diet is appropriately named because of its long-term effects. Eating too much animal flesh, fat, oil, and sugar, and too few

---

Case Study

Case Study, Part 2

The patient decides to go willingly into the ambulance. The officer joins you for the transport. Next you begin your patient interview and assessment. The patient confirms that he tried to kill himself; he denies having difficulty breathing, chest pain, dizziness, nausea, or vomiting. He was in the vehicle with the engine running for approximately 20 minutes. He takes no medications and has no allergies, and he confirms that he has been up all night drinking and planning the attempt. He allows you to administer oxygen by nonrebreathing mask and to listen to his lung sounds and obtain vital signs. There is no evidence of physical injury, but the patient appears exhausted.

Focused Physical Assessment

Recording time
10 minutes

Skin signs
Warm, dry, good color

Other signs
Breath sounds are clear.
Speech is clear and appropriate.
Body language is nonthreatening.

Vital Signs

Pulse rate/quality
74 beats/min, regular, strong

Blood pressure
122/62 mm Hg

Respiratory rate/depth
18 breaths/min, good effort

Diagnostic Tools

Electrocardiogram
Normal sinus rhythm

SpO2
100%

Blood glucose level
134 mg/dL

Question 4: What is the role of hormones in the stress reaction?

Question 5: What is the role of the immune system during a stress reaction?

CASE STUDY

---

complex carbohydrates, such as fresh vegetables and fruits, whole grains, and legumes, contributes to the development of degenerative disease. These include the major killers such as heart disease, diabetes, cancer, obesity, and strokes. It also includes a host of problematic conditions such as constipation, hemorrhoids, gout, osteoporosis, and tooth decay. According to the US Surgeon General's *Report on Nutrition and Health*, diet-related diseases account for over two thirds of all deaths in this country. Complicating the paramedic's diet are such variables as frequently rushed or interrupted

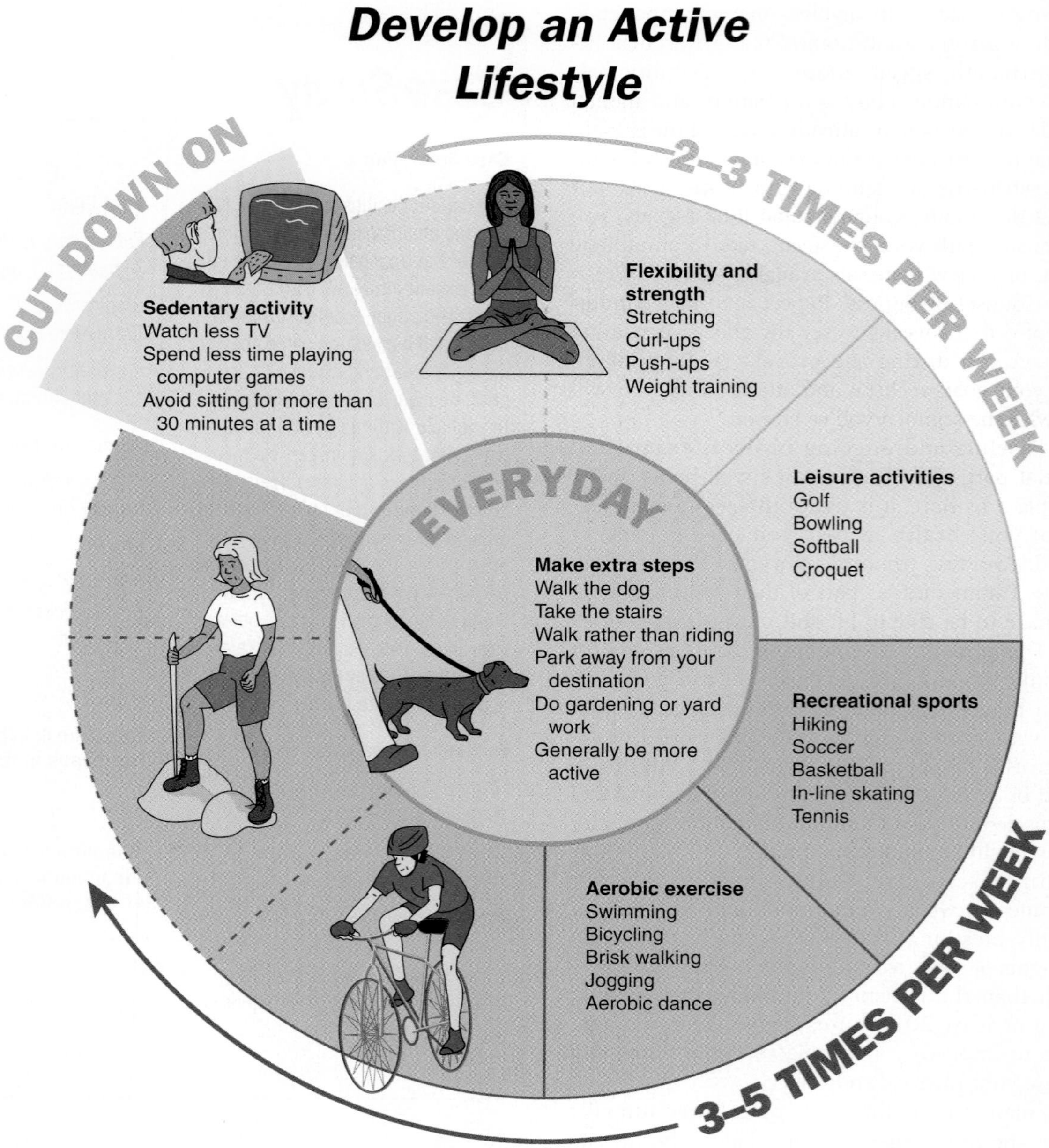

Develop an Active Lifestyle

CUT DOWN ON

Sedentary activity
Watch less TV
Spend less time playing
computer games
Avoid sitting for more than
30 minutes at a time

2-3 TIMES PER WEEK

Flexibility and strength
Stretching
Curl-ups
Push-ups
Weight training

Leisure activities
Golf
Bowling
Softball
Croquet

EVERYDAY

Make extra steps
Walk the dog
Take the stairs
Walk rather than riding
Park away from your
destination
Do gardening or yard
work
Generally be more
active

Recreational sports
Hiking
Soccer
Basketball
In-line skating
Tennis

Aerobic exercise
Swimming
Bicycling
Brisk walking
Jogging
Aerobic dance

3-5 TIMES PER WEEK

Figure 10-3 The Physical Activity Wheel. Perhaps the most important aspect of increasing physical activity is to have fun.

meals, limited choices for meals, and inadequate opportunities to prepare foods. Consider the following suggestions:

- Adjust your food planning and shopping habits so you can eat more fresh foods, stock up with healthier foods, and plan and prepare better meals.
- Pack a small cooler full of fresh fruits and vegetables that you can take with you, instead of pouring change into snack machines.

- Replace the candy or chips with popcorn or pretzels, which tend to be lower fat and lower in calories.
- Instead of stopping for greasy fast food, try some of the nutritious prepared foods offered at most moderately sized supermarkets.
- If you have to go to a fast-food restaurant, consider the alternative menu for health-conscious individuals.
- By not limiting your diet to only a few foods, you also decrease the risk that you'll miss out

on some essential vitamins and minerals. You will enjoy the food and stay with your plan.

- Begin to make small changes to your diet over an extended period of time rather than radical changes overnight. Making a slow transition is not only easier but is also more likely to work. A good start might be to cut back on fat intake; for instance, you could switch to non-fat or low-fat dairy products.

- Choose leaner cuts of meat.

- Make snacks and desserts an occasional treat instead of a regular event.

- Eat less at every meal, by leaving a little food on your plate or not taking seconds.

The Body Needs Plenty of Rest

Paramedics often have more than one job and work overtime shifts. Studies have shown that many of the automobile collisions we respond to are caused by drivers falling asleep at the wheel. The same impact of decreased amounts of sleep can affect the paramedic. Decreased amounts of sleep and irregular sleep periods are common and can cause problems such as increased fatigue and decreased alertness and contribute to poor decision making. Being a good paramedic requires sharp assessment skills and the ability to make rapid treatment decisions. If you report to work sleepy or groggy, patient care may suffer.

Preventing Disease in the Paramedic

When you are in good physical condition, your body is less likely to be susceptible to illness because your immune system will work better to protect you. You will have more energy and not tire as easily as those who are not in good physical condition. Your attitude in general will be more positive. Although paramedics care for people who are injured, more often they care for patients who are ill. If you are not in good health, you may become ill from your patients. Going to work when you are sick (eg, cold or flu symptoms) could potentially make your patients sick or worsen their condition. Remember that patients who are very young, very old, or who have preexisting medical conditions may have an already depressed immune system. Making sure your immunizations are up to date is a very important part of disease prevention for the paramedic. Keep up-to-date records of the shots you have been given. The following are guidelines for seven vaccines that are recommended for routine use:

- DPT – Diphtheria, pertussis (whooping cough), and tetanus. After the primary immunization in childhood, adults should receive tetanus and diphtheria boosters about every 10 years.

Case Study

Case Study, Part 3

En route to the hospital, you explain to the patient why you are going to draw blood samples and start an IV and what he can expect after arriving at the hospital. Your patient does not like the idea of going to the hospital, but he remains cooperative.

After starting the IV, you reassess his mental status and ABCs and obtain serial vital signs, all of which remain nearly the same as the baseline values.

Ongoing Assessment

Recording time
20 minutes

Appearance
Exhausted

Mental status
Alert, cooperative, and depressed

Vital Signs

Unchanged

Question 6: List some examples of actions that may trigger the stress response.

Question 7: List some emotional and physical signs and symptoms of stress.

CASE STUDY

Case Study

Case Study, Part 4

Completion of Case Study

This case was a behavioral emergency as well as a medical emergency. This patient has experienced a negative response (stress), which has induced physical and mental tension. The disturbance of emotional balance has led to maladaptive behavior and impaired functioning. Apparently this led to the suicide attempt (behavioral emergency) by carbon monoxide poisoning (medical emergency).

In carbon monoxide poisoning, the gas competes for receptor sites on the hemoglobin molecules at a rate 200 times greater than oxygen. The toxic-

ity of carbon monoxide poisoning varies with the length of exposure and the concentration inhaled, and the respiratory and circulatory rates. Symptoms will vary with the percentage of carboxyhemoglobin in the blood and may include dyspnea, headache, confusion, vertigo, dilated pupils, seizures, and coma.

Fortunately in this case the lack of any symptoms of carbon monoxide poisoning is a good sign. However, the patient did attempt suicide and is in need of psychiatric and emotional evaluation and care.

CASE STUDY

- Measles – This disease can be more severe in young adults than in children. It is recommended that anyone born after 1956 who did not receive live measles vaccine after age 1 year and has no documented history of measles infection should receive a single dose of measles vaccine. If you are uncertain about your history of measles, a blood test can determine if you have had the infection.

- Rubella – The objective of immunizing adults against rubella (German measles) is to prevent spread of infection to the developing fetus. If the disease is contracted in early pregnancy, fetal infection can occur in 80% of cases. Therefore, routine immunization of adults is recommended.

- Influenza – Each fall between September and November you should consider getting your flu shot. It markedly reduces the complications and death rate due to influenza, especially in older patients. Annual immunization is recommended for health care providers and those with any type of chronic medical problems, such as heart or lung disease, and for everyone older than 65 years. Adverse reactions or side effects to this vaccine have been infrequent in the last few years.

- Pneumonia vaccine – The pneumonia vaccine protects recipients from about 90% of the types of pneumonia currently active in this country.

- Hepatitis B vaccine – Hepatitis B, or serum hepatitis, is associated with an inflammation of the liver. It is commonly found in intravenous drug abusers, homosexuals, and among household members and sexual partners of people who have hepatitis. It can also occur in health care workers because of their increased exposure to blood and blood products. Paramedics are required by OSHA to receive this vaccination as part of their baseline or ongoing physical exam. The vaccine is synthetic, has very few reported side effects, and may be given during pregnancy.

- Chicken pox – Chicken pox is a standard immunization for children and recommended for paramedics who have not had the disease. Although it is relatively new, very few side effects have been reported.

Paramedic Stress: To Be Managed and Not Eliminated

Stress is an unavoidable part of everyday living. In fact, if we do not feel stress, we are probably not participating in mainstream activity. Unfortunately, stress contributes to quite a few medical problems (eg., headaches, ulcers, hypertension, colitis, skin problems, and even heart disease). Although the symptoms of stress vary widely, it is important to realize that if they are ignored they will continue to wear down the body and eventually cause damage that cannot be reversed. The best way to manage stress is to first identify its cause in your life and then look for more positive ways to interpret stressful situations. Two people in the same kind of situation can define and experience that situation quite differently; one may see it as a threat, while the other sees it as an opportunity. Anticipate situations that lead to stress (ie, consider rehearsing the conversations you might have when dealing with the family of a dying patient, the victim of rape, or a suicidal patient.) Once you are able to do this, you can plan more effectively for those inevitable situations.

A useful stress-reducing technique is to allot at least 15 minutes a day for personal quiet time. Simply relax, meditate, or pray. Slow, deep, abdominal breathing can also be very effective. Remember although we cannot totally eliminate stress from our lives, we can change the way we perceive it and the way in which we respond to it.

A Healthy Mental Attitude

Try to balance family, work, and recreation by not giving too much "weight" to only one of these components. A positive mental attitude can be a form of preventive medicine. The paramedic, who occasionally feels down, even depressed, may seem to get sick more often during these times. A person's attitude toward life has been shown to affect his or her health. People who are more cheerful and who take time to "smell the roses" have fewer problems with sickness. A cheerful outlook will not prevent the development of all disease states, but research has shown that laughter can have a curing effect. An amazing transformation takes place in people who become very sick, even to the point of near-death, and then get well again; most people who go through that experience suddenly find that their family relationships are more meaningful and life is more precious. It seems that the worse the illness, the more spectacular the change in attitude, and the greater the meaning of life becomes. The message here is to try to improve your outlook now in order to avoid getting sick.

So you have set your goals, you have selected a physical conditioning workout that is right for you, you have updated your health records with your physician, and you are working to improve your attitude and better manage the stress in your life. You have also considered your nutritional needs and have chosen a diet. You should be well on your way to improving your health as well as making your work as a paramedic easier and safer.

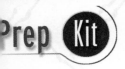

Chapter Summary

- Stress has often been called the proxy killer because it can cause diseases that ultimately lead to the patient's death.

- The general adaptation syndrome describes the body's short-term and long-term reactions to stress. The first stage, called the alarm reaction, is the immediate reaction to a stressor in which the body releases adrenaline and other psychological mechanisms to combat the stress and to stay in control. Humans exhibit a fight-or-flight reaction. The body reacts to stress first by releasing catecholamines, the most abundant of which are epinephrine (adrenaline), norepinephrine (noradrenaline), and dopamine.

- In stage two, the body adapts to the stressors it is exposed to. This is the body's way of providing long-term protection. The body secretes additional hormones that increase blood glucose levels to sustain energy and raise blood pressure. The adrenal cortex (outer covering) produces hormones called corticosteroids for this resistance reaction. If this phase continues for a prolonged period of time without periods of relaxation and rest to counterbalance the stress response, sufferers become prone to fatigue, concentration

lapses, irritability, and lethargy as the effort to sustain arousal becomes negative stress.

- The third stage, in which the body has run out of its reserve of body energy and immunity, is called exhaustion. Mental, physical, and emotional resources suffer greatly and the body experiences "adrenal exhaustion." The blood glucose levels decrease as the adrenals become depleted, leading to decreased stress tolerance, progressive mental and physical exhaustion, illness, and collapse.

- The HPA axis is a major part of the neuroendocrine system that controls reactions to stress. The HPA axis is believed to play a primary role in the body's reactions to stress, by balancing hormone releases from the adrenaline-producing adrenal medulla. Increased cortisol production exhausts the stress mechanism and interferes with serotonin, leading to fatigue and depression.

- The lifestyle of a paramedic in a busy EMS system can be very stressful. For this reason, it is especially important for paramedics to take steps to maintain good health and reduce unnecessary stress.

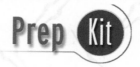

Vital Vocabulary

alarm reaction The first stage of the general adaptation syndrome, which is the body's immediate reaction to the stressor.

catecholamines Chemical compounds derived from the amino acid tyrosine, which acts as a hormone or neurotransmitter.

exhaustion stage The third and final stage of the general adaptation syndrome in which the body's resistance to stress is gradually reduced or may quickly collapse.

general adaptation syndrome A description of the body's short-term and long-term reactions to stress.

Hassles Scale Developed by Richard Lazarus, a scale of events or daily interruptions with the environment that are essentially negative.

health A state of complete physical, mental, and social well-being. Health is the vital principle that enables us to meet and overcome the challenges of the day.

hypothalamic-pituitary-adrenal (HPA) axis A major part of the neuroendocrine system that controls reactions to stress. It is the mechanism for a set of interactions among glands, hormones, and parts of the mid-brain that mediate the general adaptation syndrome.

life-change units (LCUs) First described in the life chart theory by Adolph Meyer, LCUs are used to provide a weighted scale based on stress-producing events in a person's life.

resistance stage The second stage of the general adaption syndrome, which is the body's attempt to adapt to the stressors it is exposed to.

Case Study Answers

Question 1: What is stress?

Answer: Stress is defined as a factor that induces bodily or mental tension. Stress is a natural and necessary emotion and can be good (eustress) or bad (distress).

Question 2: What is general adaptation syndrome and what are its three stages?

Answer: General adaptation syndrome is a nonspecific defense system of the body initiated by stress. The three phases of the syndrome are the alarm reaction, which is analogous to the fight-or-flight response; the stage of resistance, which is an adaptive phase; and the stage of exhaustion, in which the body systems become overwhelmed and begin to fail.

Question 3: What is the role of cortisol in a stress response?

Answer: Any type of stress can cause the release of cortisol from the adrenal gland. Cortisol affects metabolism in the following ways: (1) it decreases protein reserves, (2) it increases blood glucose concentration and impairs the utilization of glucose by peripheral tissues, and (3) it permits mobilization of fatty acids by epinephrine and the growth hormone. Continual increased cortisol production exhausts the stress mechanism, leading to fatigue, depression, and a depressed immune system.

Question 4: What is the role of hormones in the stress reaction?

Answer: Two types of hormones are released during the stress reaction: peptides (epinephrine and glucagon) and corticosteroids (cortisol). Epinephrine and glucagons stimulate the sympathetic nervous system, leading to various effects including an increase in blood glucose. Cortisol works as described in the answer to question 3. The combined effect is that the body is better equipped to handle stress by making more nutrients available and the body is better able to utilize them.

Question 5: What is the role of the immune system during a stress reaction?

Answer: The quick and short-term response is the fight-or-flight response, which triggers catecholamine release. This leads to increased levels of available white blood cells. Long-term or chronic distress and the resultant neuroendocrine activation can induce immune system suppression.

Question 6: List some examples of actions that may trigger the stress response.

Answer: Some examples include poor health or nutrition, the loss of a loved one or something of value, an injury or threat of an injury to the body, and ineffective coping mechanism.

Question 7: List some emotional and physical signs and symptoms of stress.

Answer: Physical signs of stress can include chest pain or tightness, heart palpitations, cardiac rhythm disturbances, difficulty breathing, nausea, vomiting, sweating, flushed skin, sleep disturbances, muscle aches, or headache. Emotional signs and symptoms of stress may include panic reactions, fear, anger, denial, and feeling overwhelmed.

Photo Credits

Chapter 2

Figure 2-2 Part A inset © Fred Hossler/Visuals Unlimited. Part B inset © David M. Phillips/Visuals Unlimited

Figure 2-3 Parts A and C © Ed Reschke/Visuals Unlimited. Part B © M.I. Walker/Science Source/Photo Researchers, Inc.

Figure 2-4 Part A © David M. Phillips/Visuals Unlimited

Figure 2-9 Courtesy L. Crowley

Chapter 3

Figure 3-1 Courtesy L. Crowley

Figure 3-2 Part B © Don W. Fawcett/Visuals Unlimited

Figure 3-5 Part B © David M. Phillips/Visuals Unlimited

Figure 3-6 Part C © G. Musil/Visuals Unlimited

Chapter 4

Figures 4-1, 4-7, 4-10, 4-17, 4-18, 4-19, and **4-20** Courtesy L. Crowley

Figure 4-15 © Nils Meilvang/AP Photos

Chapter 5

Figures 5-5, 5-6, 5-9, 5-10, 5-13, 5-16, 5-17, and **5-18** Courtesy L. Crowley

Figure 5-14 Data from National Institute of Diabetes and Digestive and Kidney Diseases (NIDDK), NIH. Washington, DC; and Enattah, N.S., Sahi, T., Savilahti, E., et al. Identification of a variant associated with adult-type hypolactasia. *Nat. Genet.* 2002; 30(2):223–237

Chapter 6

Figure 6-1 Courtesy of Dey, L.P.

Figures 6-3, 6-4, and **6-5** Courtesy L. Crowley

Chapter 7

Figures 7-2, 7-10, and **7-11** Courtesy L. Crowley

Figure 7-4 © R. Calentine/Visuals Unlimited

Figure 7-5 © W. Johnson/Visuals Unlimited

Chapter 8

Figures 8-1, 8-2, and **8-7** Courtesy L. Crowley

Figure 8-3 © David M. Phillips/Visuals Unlimited

Chapter 9

Figure 9-3 Courtesy L. Crowley

Figure 9-4 Courtesy Dr. Robert A. Marcus

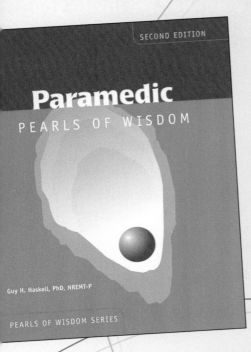
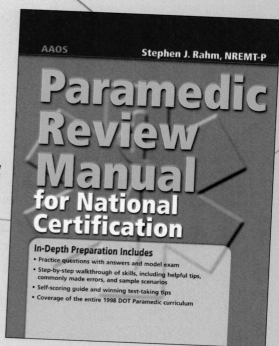

Did you know that Jones and Bartlett (J&B) already publishes an extensive line of training materials for Paramedic courses? We invite you to consider the other paramedic texts J&B already offers, including:

AAOS PARAMEDIC SERIES

Written for paramedics by paramedics, this series uses a case-based approach to help future paramedics develop analytical skills, while learning the content of airway management, anatomy and physiology, and pathophysiology.

Paramedic: Pathophysiology
American Academy of Orthopaedic Surgeons (AAOS), Bob Elling, MPA, REMT-P, Kirsten M. Elling, BS, REMT-P, Mikel A. Rothenberg, MD
ISBN: 0-7637-3765-8 • $47.95 (Sugg. US List) • Paperback • 320 pages • © 2006

Paramedic: Anatomy & Physiology
American Academy of Orthopaedic Surgeons (AAOS), Bob Elling, MPA, REMT-P, Kirsten M. Elling, BS, REMT-P, Mikel A. Rothenberg, MD
ISBN: 0-7637-3792-5 • $47.95 (Sugg. US List) • Paperback • 320 Pages • © 2004

Paramedic: Airway Management
American Academy of Orthopaedic Surgeons (AAOS), Gregg Margolis, MS, NREMT-P
ISBN: 0-7637-1327-9 • $47.95 (Sugg. US List) • Paperback • 332 Pages • © 2004

12-LEAD SERIES

Become a fully advanced interpreter of ECGs with this series! Using hundreds of four-color graphics and full-size rhythm strips, these texts help students with little or no knowledge of electrocardiology become adept at reading and interpreting ECGs.

12-Lead ECG: The Art of Interpretation
Tomas B. Garcia, MD, Neil Holtz, BS, EMT-P
ISBN: 0-7637-1284-1 • $49.95 (Sugg. US List) • Paperback • 536 Pages • © 2001

Introduction to 12-Lead ECG: The Art of Interpretation
Tomas B. Garcia, MD, Neil Holtz, BS, EMT-P
ISBN: 0-7637-1961-7 • $39.95 (Sugg. US List) • Paperback • 236 Pages • © 2003

Arrhythmia Recognition: The Art of Interpretation
Tomas B. Garcia, MD, Geoffrey T. Miller, NREMT-P
ISBN: 0-7637-2246-4 • $64.95 (Sugg. US List) • Paperback • 633 Pages • © 2004

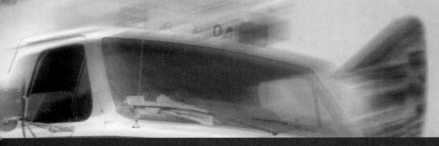
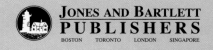